HEALING HERBS

How to Grow, Store, and Maximize Their Medicinal Power

SECOND EDITION

DEDE CUMMINGS *and* ALYSSA HOLMES

Foreword by Barbara Fahs

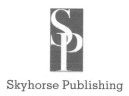

Skyhorse Publishing

Skyhorse Publishing books may be purchased in bulk at special discounts for sales promotion, corporate gifts, fund-raising, or educational purposes. Special editions can also be created to specifications. For details, contact the Special Sales Department, Skyhorse Publishing, 307 West 36th Street, 11th Floor, New York, NY 10018 or info@skyhorsepublishing.com.

Skyhorse® and Skyhorse Publishing® are registered trademarks of Skyhorse Publishing, Inc.®, a Delaware corporation.

Visit our website:
www.skyhorsepublishing.com.

Please follow our publisher Tony Lyons on Instagram @tonylyonsisuncertain

10 9 8 7 6 5 4 3 2 1

Library of Congress Cataloging-in-Publication Data is available on file.

Cover design by Jane Sheppard
Cover photos by Abigail Gehring, iStock

Print ISBN: 978-1-5107-7877-1
eBook ISBN: 978-1-5107-1611-7

Printed in China

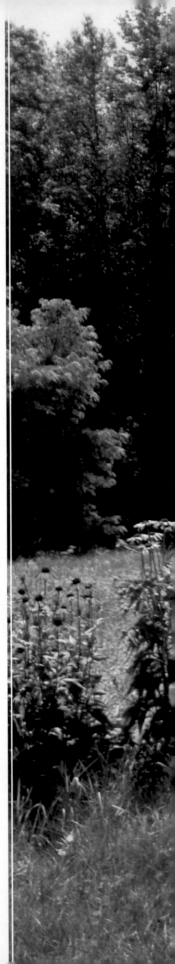

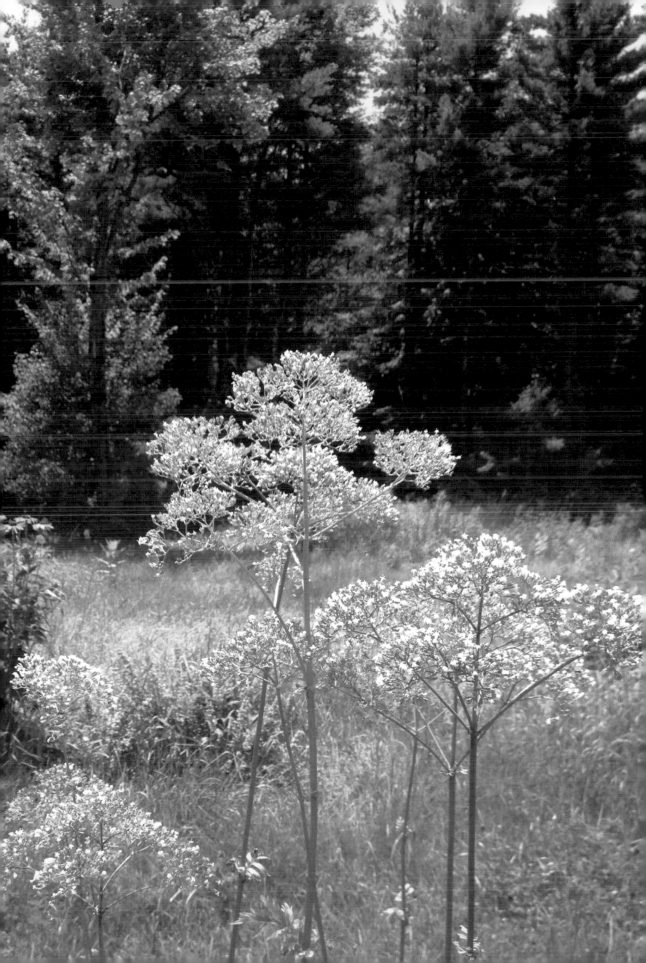

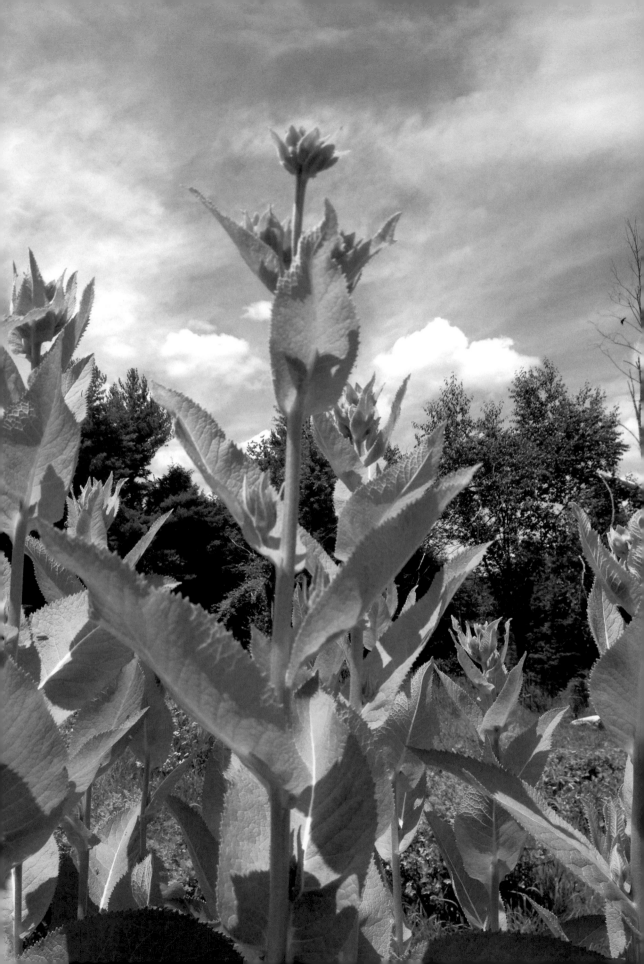

CONTENTS

Foreword by Barbara Fahs   vii

Introduction   ix
Why grow medicinal herbs in your backyard

Meet the Plants   1
Getting to know your herbal allies

Cultivating the Medicinal Garden   65
*Design, location, choosing the herbs to grow, planting,
and maintenance*

  Implementing the Medicinal
    Herb Garden   75
  Testing, Soil Types, and Amending
    Your Soil   81
  Planting Your Garden   83

Urban Medicinal Gardening   93
*Growing in small spaces, containers, windowsills,
and on rooftops*

From Harvest to Storage   97
*When to harvest, how to harvest, drying methods,
and storage*

  Harvesting   99
  Drying   101
  Storage   103

**Simple Herbal Medicines
& Home Remedies   105**
*How to make teas (infusions and decoctions), syrups,
dental health recipes, tinctures, powders (capsules,
pills, and poultices), oils, salves, liniments, baths,
sachets, dream pillows, and smudges*

Conclusion   129

Appendices
  Appendix 1   131
    Properties and Actions of Herbs   131
  Appendix 2   133
    Additional Herbal Remedies   133
  Appendix 3   143
    Freezing Fresh Herbs   143
  Appendix 4   145
    Dosages   145
  Appendix 5   146
    Collecting Herbs in the Wild   146
  Appendix 6   148
    Cooking with Herbs   148
    Recipes   151
  Appendix 7   155
    Herbal Cocktails   155
  Appendix 8   156
    The Healing Power of Mushrooms   156
    A Few Edible and Medicinal
      Mushroom Profiles   157

Resources   159
  Companies/Organizations   159
  Books   160

About the Authors   163

Photo Credits   167

Index   168

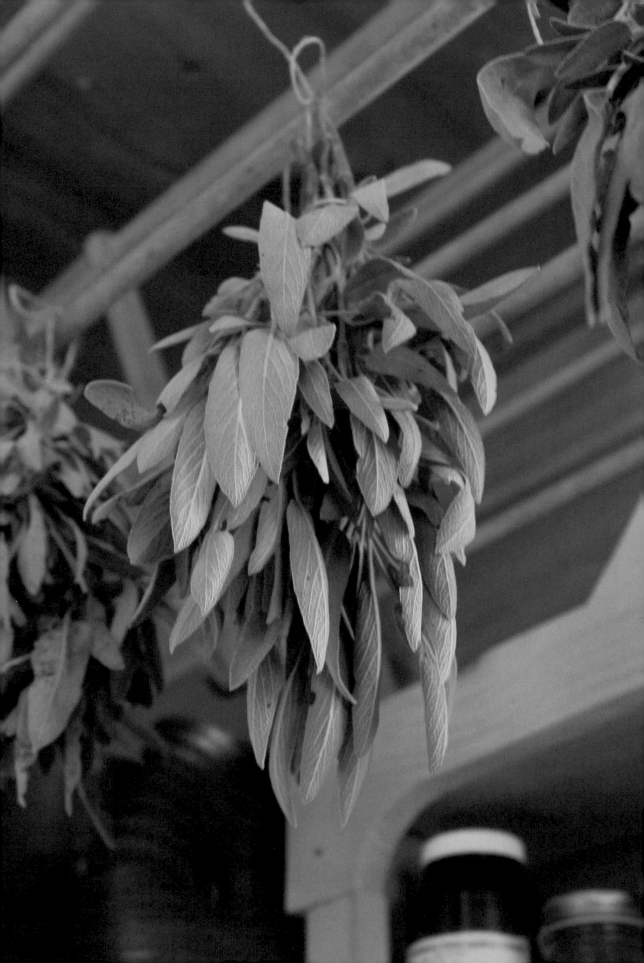

FOREWORD

Before this book, you needed several different reference sources to put together all of the useful information about how to grow and use medicinal plants. From starting a garden, to planting, to weed and insect control, to harvesting and preserving the plants, to making simple, effective medicines from them, the authors cover everything you need to get started on a lifetime of learning and health. And they make it fun! Their personable approach to the various subjects just makes the reader want to read more.

Alyssa and Dede have synthesized valuable information about 24 very special medicinal plants and have included instructions for growing or collecting them in a clear, simple, straightforward manner. Focusing on a core group of plants, as the authors have done, helps greatly to clarify the mystifying plethora of plants that can be used as medicine. The concepts of "wonderful weeds" and native plants are important topics that I always stress in my own classes, garden tours and writing. If only everyone would learn to look at our plant heritage with these eyes! Some of my very favorite "weeds" are covered here, so it's great that more people will learn about them through this book. Think of the "weeds" you have struggled to remove from your lawn—dandelion, plantain, red clover, and others—and you might then rethink your eradication of them.

Growing organically, without poisons and chemicals, is vital when growing medicinals. If we want to heal ourselves with Mother Nature's bounty, we must participate in her natural processes rather than fight them, attempting to control the physical world, as we humans so often attempt to do.

Although the climate and gardening conditions where I live in Hawaii are very different from the US mainland (believe it or not, the mints do not survive long-term here!), I have had much experience growing many of the plants the authors describe when I lived in Northern California from 1971 until 1998. Their gardening advice is sound and is presented in an easy-to-understand way. The important thing I have learned about growing medicinal herbs is that they grow best when they grow where they want to grow. I always tell visitors to my garden, "the plants don't need us, but we need the plants." This basic philosophy is echoed in the pages of this book, and the authors have done a good job of communicating the importance of letting the plants do their own thing. Very little fussing, fretting, and fertilizing are needed for this category of plants!

Appendix 1 includes a succinct list of the properties that medicinal plants can contain. Along with simple definitions and good examples of plants that have each property, this quick reference will help all readers to learn the sometimes confusing terms and will enable them to better design their own unique formulas that will serve their special needs exceptionally well.

I am confident that readers of this book will become inspired to plant a garden that contains at least a few medicinals. They will change your life for the better, in many wonderful ways.

—Barbara Fahs
Author of *Super Simple Guide to Creating Hawaiian Gardens* and the "Healthful Herbalist" newspaper column; teacher of workshops, including the Home Herbalist Certification Series.

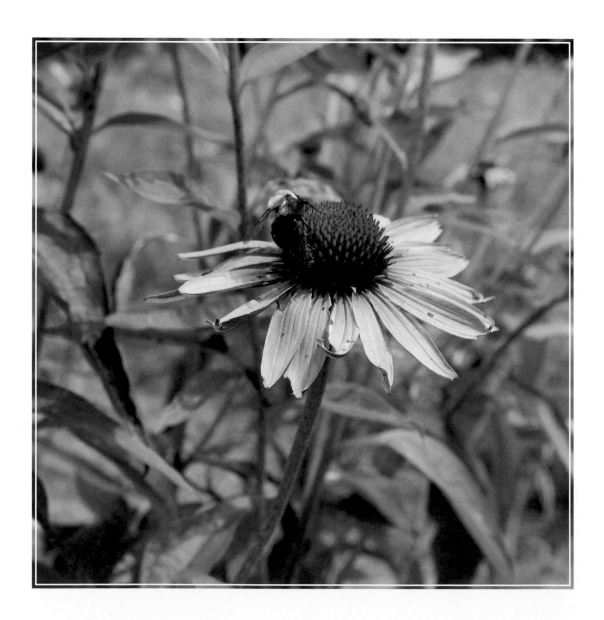

INTRODUCTION

People have used plants as medicine since the beginning of time. Every culture around the world has or has lost a relationship to the plants of the region, whether wild or cultivated. These healing plants have served our species well. There was once a time, in the not too distant past, when most people had some knowledge of plants to heal themselves, and in every village a person of more expertise on treating serious conditions.

Today we are focused on so many different things in our busy lives, and most of us have come to depend on systems of medicine that are outside of ourselves. We have forgotten how to take care of ourselves, prevent illness, and treat common ailments when they arise. We may be fearful when something is off balance, in turn running to the nearest hospital or pharmacy. We have forgotten how to grow and prepare the simplest of medicines to treat colds, flus, fevers, and headaches, promote sleep, and so on. We can get this knowledge back for vibrant well-being. We can grow a small number of herbs, take a small amount of time in our lives, and have security in knowing that we can heal.

Let us be empowered to take at least some of our health into our own hands; it is we who know our bodies from the inside out! Growing a small number of medicinal herbs and/or making some simple medicines is a wonderful place to start. By doing this, we start to remember our connection with these allies, this support system that lies within the earth, and our own optimal health.

Growing and working with herbs is easy, and super fun! Herbs are wonderful "weeds" that, when put into the right environment, will grow big and strong and full. They want to spread, take over, and multiply, which is great, when they are planted where we want them! The task becomes pruning, thinning, pulling, and harvesting. Once herbs are established and growing in your yard, there is more abundance each year, rarely a worry of shortage. They are flexible and hardy to many growing conditions, oftentimes even extreme or harsh weather. The key is to choose plants that are generally suited to your area, and the ones we have chosen for this book are very common and easy to grow in most areas. Perennial herbs for the most part are the focus in this book, as they will proliferate for many years, so that establishing your garden is a one-time endeavor.

Herbs are effective medicine, not only for us, but for the garden. They serve as pest control, and they heal the earth where it may have been stripped or polluted. Incorporating them into our lives enriches us by soothing or stimulating

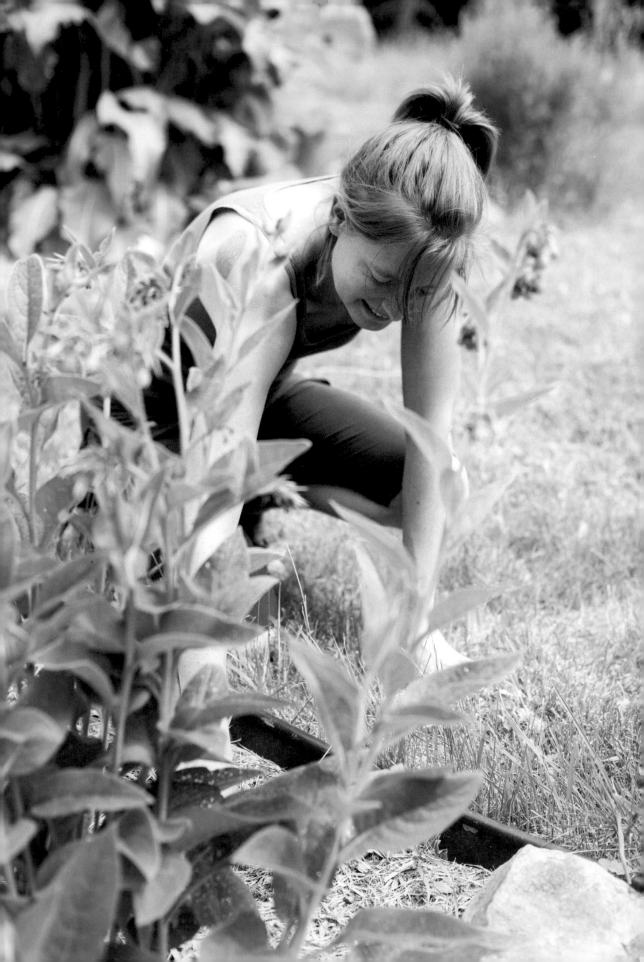

the senses and helping us feel better when sick.

This book will teach you step by step how to prepare the soil, plant the herbs, and maintain the garden in your backyard. We will also talk about alternative ways to grow herbs if you do not have a yard, as well as the abundant wild medicinal plants in fields, forests, and even urban areas.

* * *

We have chosen **thirty** herbs to cover in detail—the properties, benefits, uses, and growing methods of each one, preparing you with information to better know them, and in turn make medicine from them. There are so many more than these thirty, but learning about these will give you a solid foundation from which to expand your knowledge if you choose.

Beyond the growing, there is the harvesting, processing, and making of simple medicines for you and your family. Bringing the herbs inside and filling your home with the herbs' beauty and aroma is amazing and healing in itself.

Then we create! Create remedies for common ailments, teas, salves, extracts, pillows, oils, powders, liniments, and baths. Each year you will form more and more of a rhythm with this process—from the backyard into the kitchen and home pharmacy. You will become your own healer for many things you once relied on others for.

In the following pages you will find profiles for each of the herbs and basic garden layouts and plans.

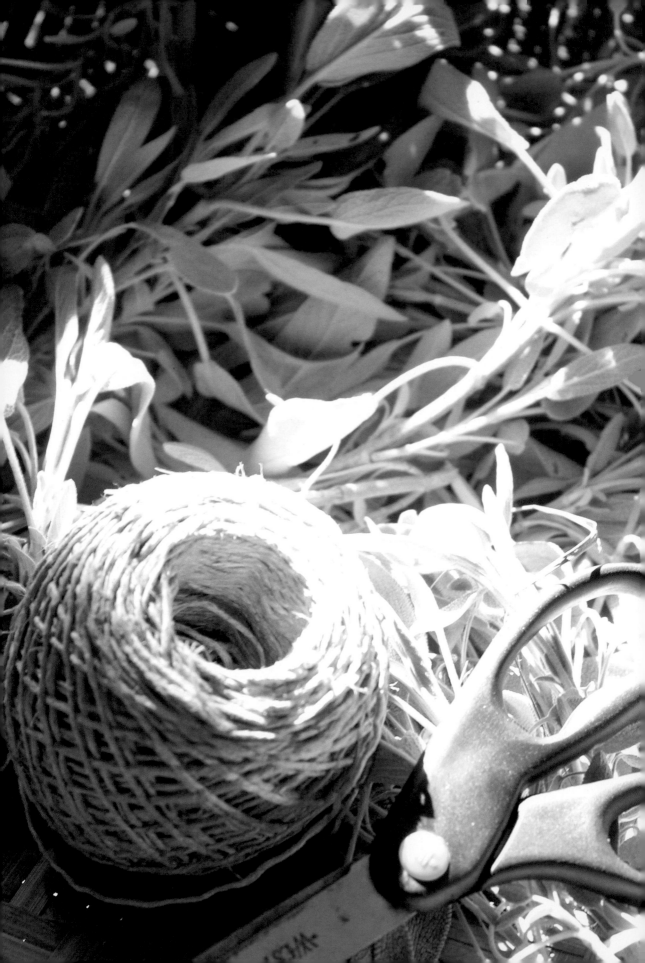

HEALING
HERBS

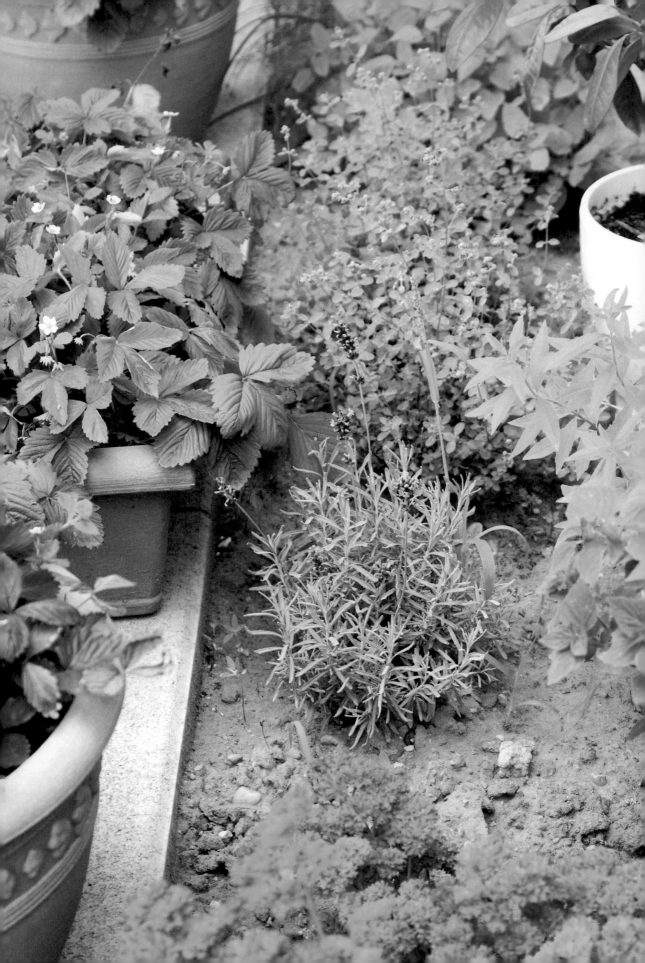

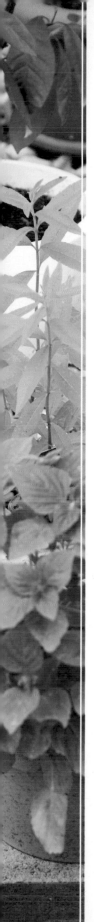

MEET THE PLANTS

Long before we had electronic databases or comprehensive scientific tomes filled with information about herbs, humans knew and understood the healing power of plants. I am convinced that this knowing came from an intrinsic sense of relationship with the plants, not simply a trial-and-error process as we often postulate.

—Rosemary Gladstar, *Family Herbal:
A Guide to Living Life with Energy, Health, and Vitality*

Getting to know plants is a rewarding process. It is also never ending. Plants are as complex as humans, adapting to the environment they are put in, struggling, thriving, producing, and giving.

Plants give us so much in the way of health and beauty. They offer a plethora of gifts from the earth and lessons to learn. They are filled with minerals and vitamins, and each one comes with its own unique profile of properties and actions, which help heal our every ailment, lift us up when we're down, and soothe our senses.

Herbs are our allies, and once your eyes are open to their world and you start to use them for your food and medicine, life will become all the better. It feels so good to take your health into your own hands when appropriate (remember that serious health considerations need professional guidance). There is so much we can do with herbs to help prevent serious illness, and so many ways herbs can help us to feel enlivened, healthy, and whole.

On the pages that follow are profiles of thirty plants we have chosen. These are commonly and easily cultivated in your backyard, windowsill, deck, or rooftop, or they are common medicinal weeds.

The list of useful medicinal herbs in this world is endless, too many for any book to cover, so we thought we would focus in with a magnifying glass on some that we think are fabulous, and some of our personal favorites!

The thirty plants in this section are incorporated into many of the recipes in the simple home remedies section (see page 105), along with other herbs and ingredients.

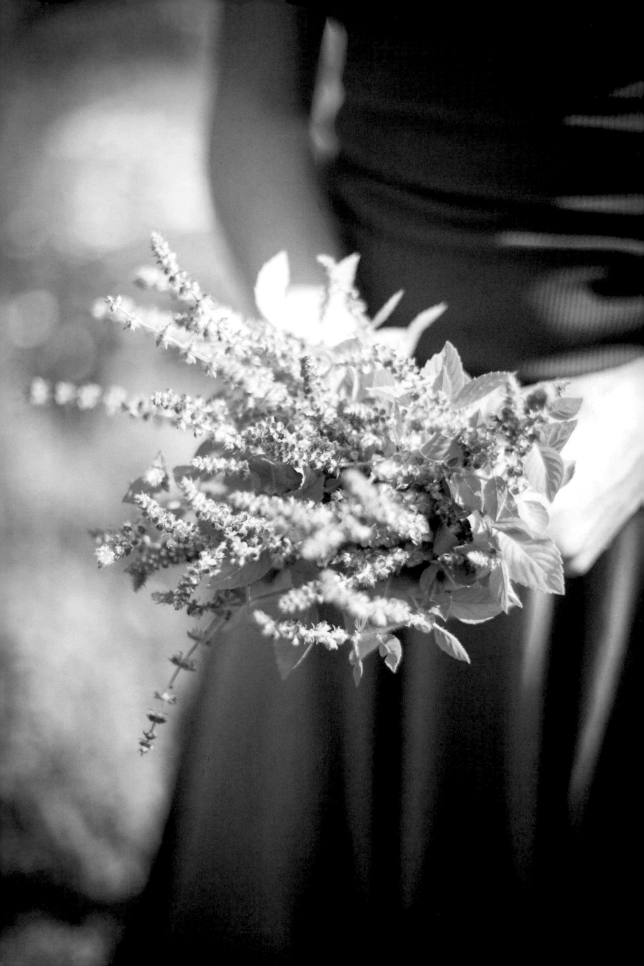

Healing Herbs

- Astragalus
- Boneset
- Burdock
- Calendula
- Chamomile
- Coltsfoot
- Comfrey
- Dandelion
- Echinacea
- Elder
- Feverfew
- Garlic
- Goldenrod
- Lavender
- Lemon balm
- Motherwort
- Mugwort
- Mullein
- Nettle
- Peppermint
- Plantain
- Red clover
- Red raspberry
- Rose
- Sage
- Self-heal
- St. John's wort
- Valerian
- Yarrow
- Yellow dock

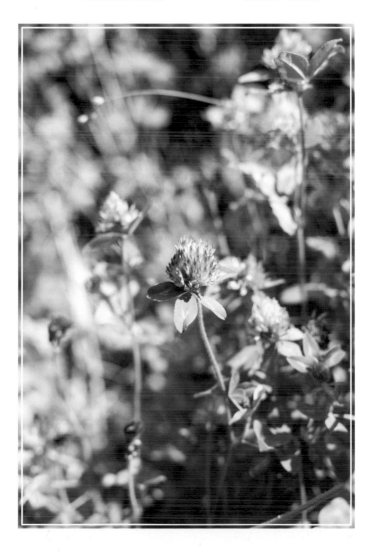

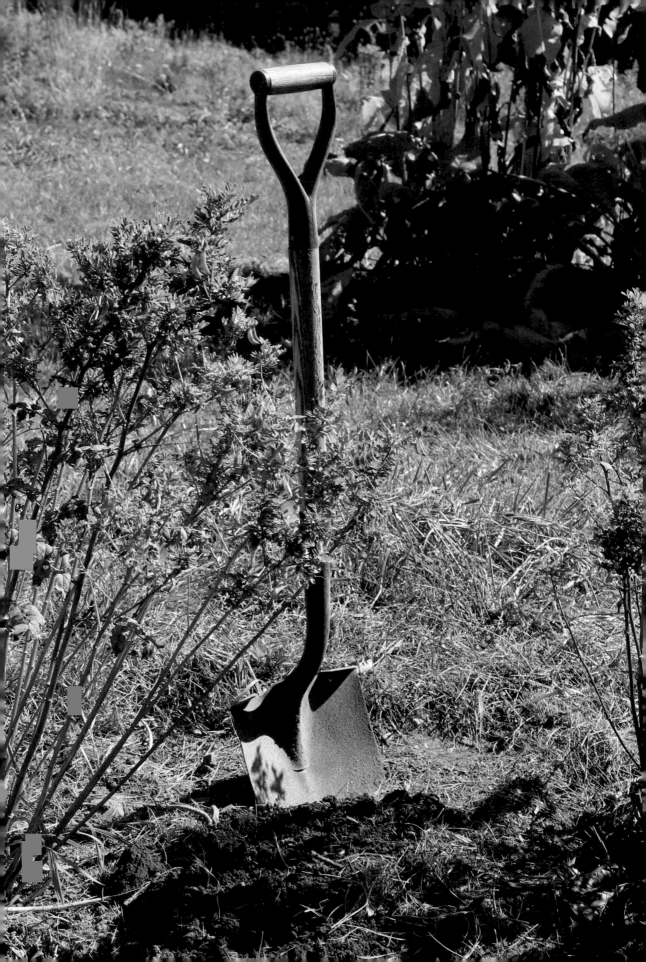

Astragalus
Astragalus membranaceus

Parts used: Root

Properties/Actions: Adaptogenic, immunomodulating, cardiotonic, antitumor, diuretic, hypotensive, anti-inflammatory.

Benefits: Strengthens the body as a general immune tonic, especially if taken over long periods of time. Balances the energy of all organs, increases energy, supports digestion.

Astragalus is very beneficial for any individuals suffering from wasting or exhausting diseases.

Suggested uses: Tincture, decoction, capsules.

Growing, harvesting, and wild crafting tips and specifics: Perennial. Grows well in full sun or partial shade. Prefers dry, sandy soil. Start from divided root, or seed.

If starting from seed, freeze the seeds for 21 days, then scarify them with fine sandpaper. Start indoors in late winter, after soaking the seeds for a day or two. Transplant into the garden in spring after danger of frost.

Protect well with mulch of leaves or straw or hay for the winter.

Cautions: May be contraindicated with medicines that suppress the immune system.

In Chinese medical terms, astragalus builds up the protective chi. Imagine that there is a protective shield around your body, just below the surface of the skin, that keeps out cold and other external influences. It vitalizes the non-specific immune defenses and wards off infections. This is the protective chi, and astragalus is the premier herb in Chinese herbalism to strengthen it.

—Paul Bergner

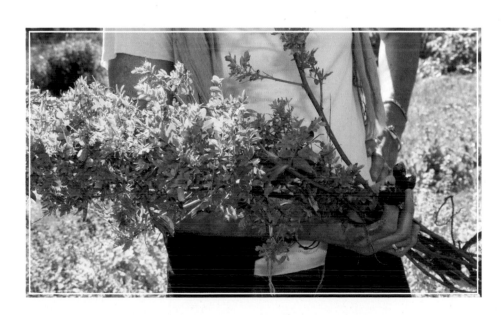

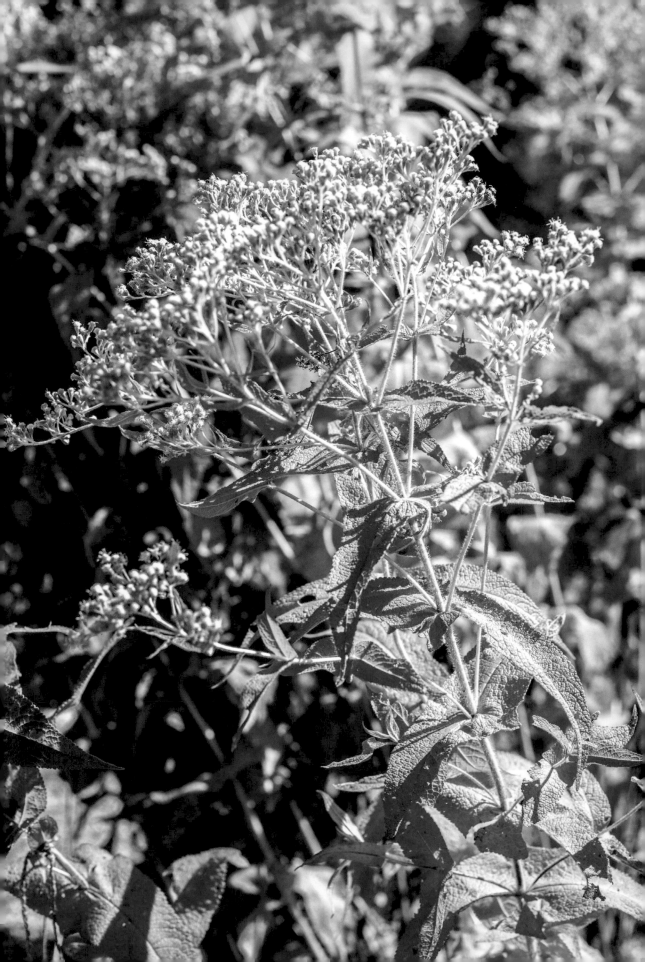

Boneset
Eupatorium perfoliatum

Parts used: Flowers, leaves, and stem

Properties/Actions: Febrifuge, diaphoretic, expectorant, laxative.

Benefits: Fevers, colds and flu, aids liver detoxification.

Suggested uses: Infusion, or tincture added to warm water.

Growing, harvesting, and wild crafting tips and specifics: Perennial. Grows big and tall, shading other plants. The best time for planting seeds is in late summer or fall. Plant your starters or divided roots, either in fall before danger of frost or in spring after the threat of frost has passed. Once established, boneset is very frost hardy.

Cautions: Can be a laxative as mentioned, so use with caution if diarrhea is present. Causes sweating (diaphoretic).

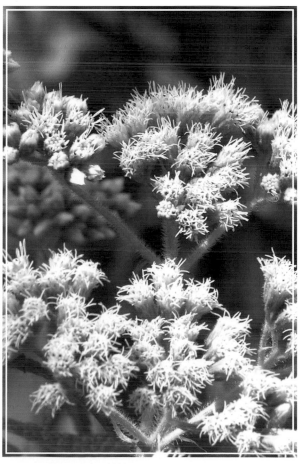

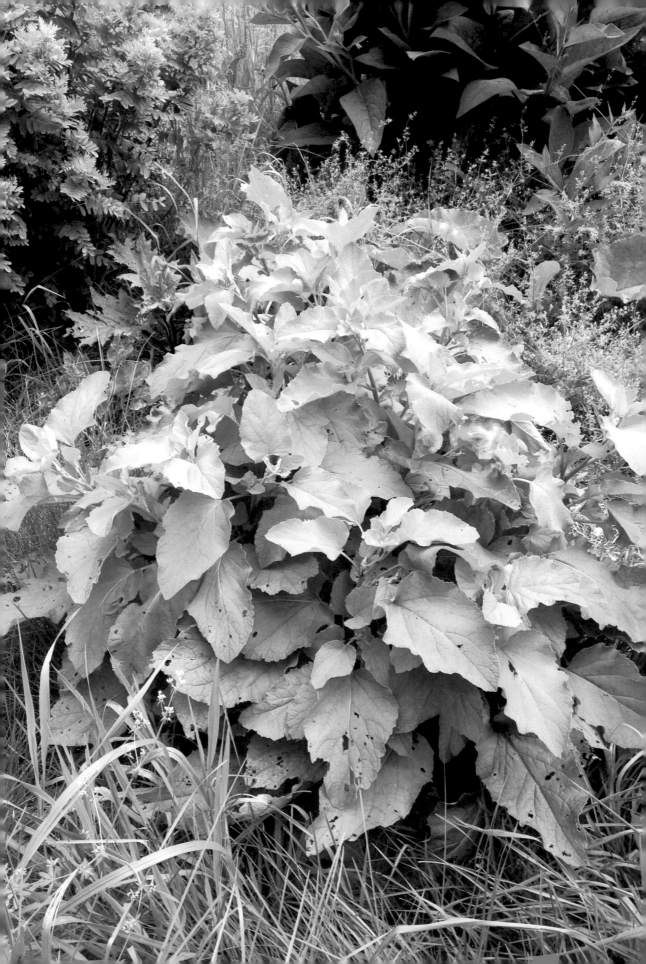

Burdock
Arctium lappa

Parts used: Root.

Properties/Actions: Alterative, antibacterial, antifungal, anti-inflammatory, diuretic, mild laxative, diaphoretic, nutritive, choleretic.

Benefits: Helps to heal skin eruptions such as acne, psoriasis, eczema, boils, carbuncles, and sties. Eases sciatica and gout, female hormonal inbalance, mastitis.

Burdock is filled with an abundance of minerals, especially iron. A valuable blood purifier, removes toxic wastes from the body, and promotes kidney function.

Great in combination with dandelion for any skin diseases.

Suggested Uses: Decoction, tincture, or eaten in soups.

Growing, harvesting, and wild crafting tips and specifics: Biennial. Grows in fields and forest edges, roadsides, and open woodlands. Thrives in poor soil. Harvest second-year roots for medicine, and first-year roots for food.

Cautions: The seed clusters—called burrs—cling to your clothing and hair!

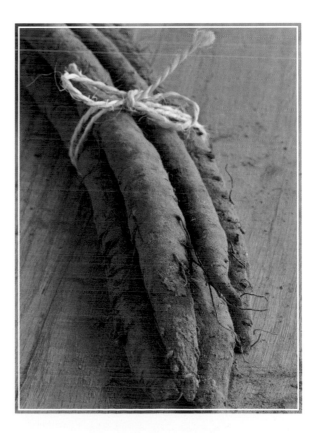

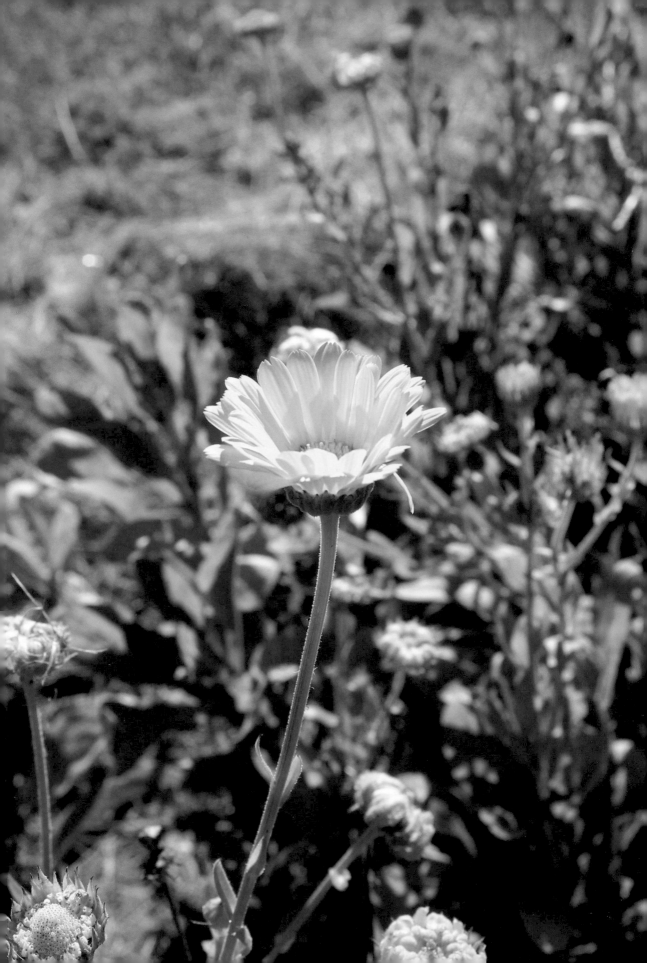

Calendula
Calendula officinalis

Parts used: Flowers.

Properties/Actions: Emollient, antiviral, anti-inflammatory, antiseptic, demulcent.

Benefits: Helps to heal cuts and scrapes, rashes, eases abdominal cramps and constipation.

Suggested uses: Tincture, infusion, herbal oil, salve.

Growing, harvesting, and wild crafting tips and specifics: Annual. Easy to start from seed directly in the garden, and will tend to self seed for following years, acting as a perennial.

Cautions: May be contraindicated during pregnancy due to aborteficient properties.

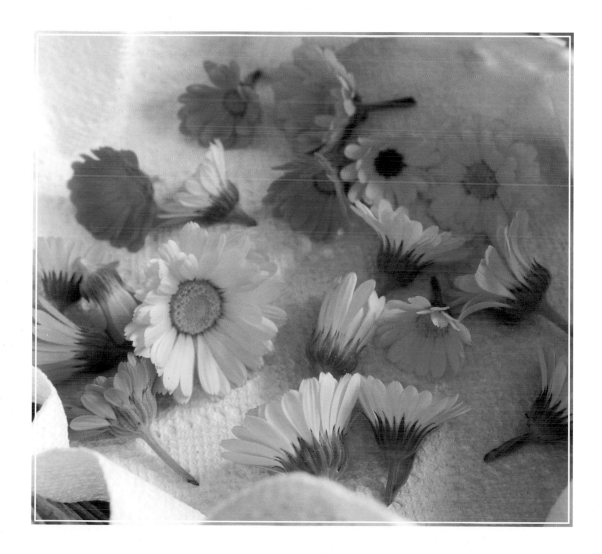

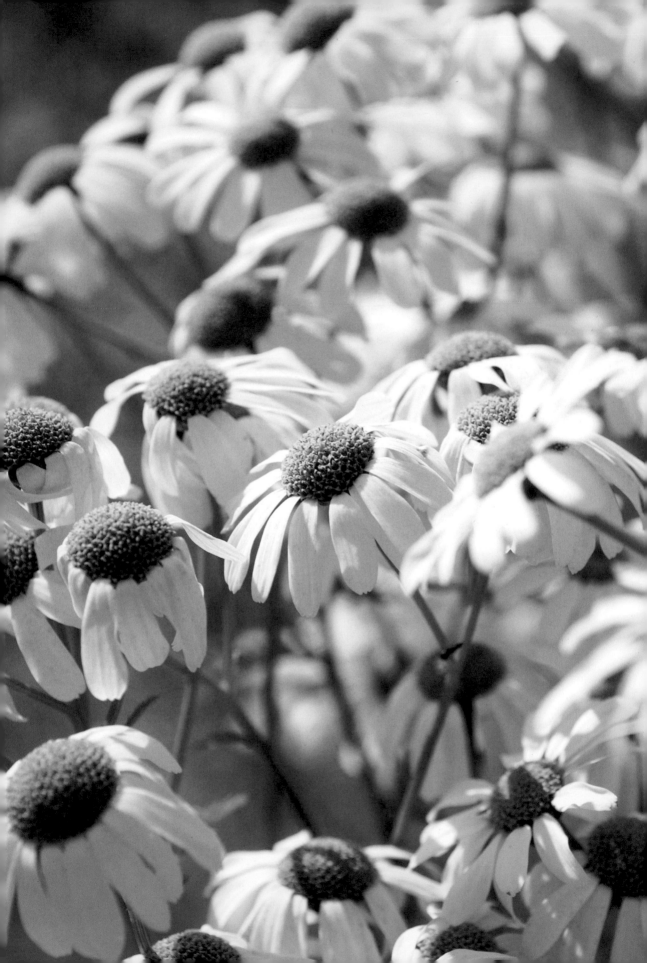

Chamomile
Matricaria recutita

Parts used: Flowers.

Properties/Actions: Antiseptic, anti-inflammatory.

Benefits: Can be used to aid in reducing inflammation, stress, and insomnia; helps with digestive problems by gently stimulating bile production. Soothing and cleansing as a compress/wash for wounds and rashes, and eye problems.

Suggested uses: Infusion, tincture, glycerite.

Growing, harvesting, and wild crafting tips and specifics: Annual. Start from seed indoors or in a greenhouse in early spring, transplant outside after danger of frost. Can be susceptible to fungi and insects in the garden, more than other herbs, so interplanting is best. There is a specific tool for efficiently harvesting the flowers of chamomile, called a chamomile rake.

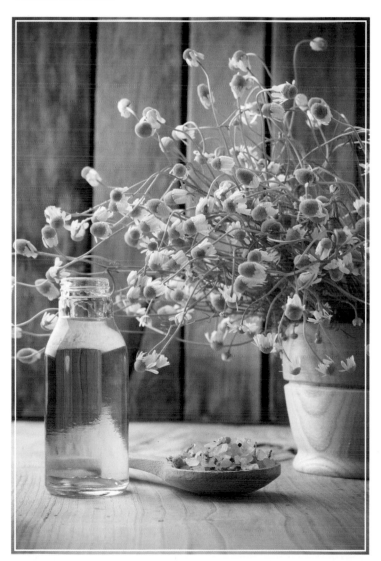

Cautions: People who have ragweed allergies may have the same reaction to chamomile.

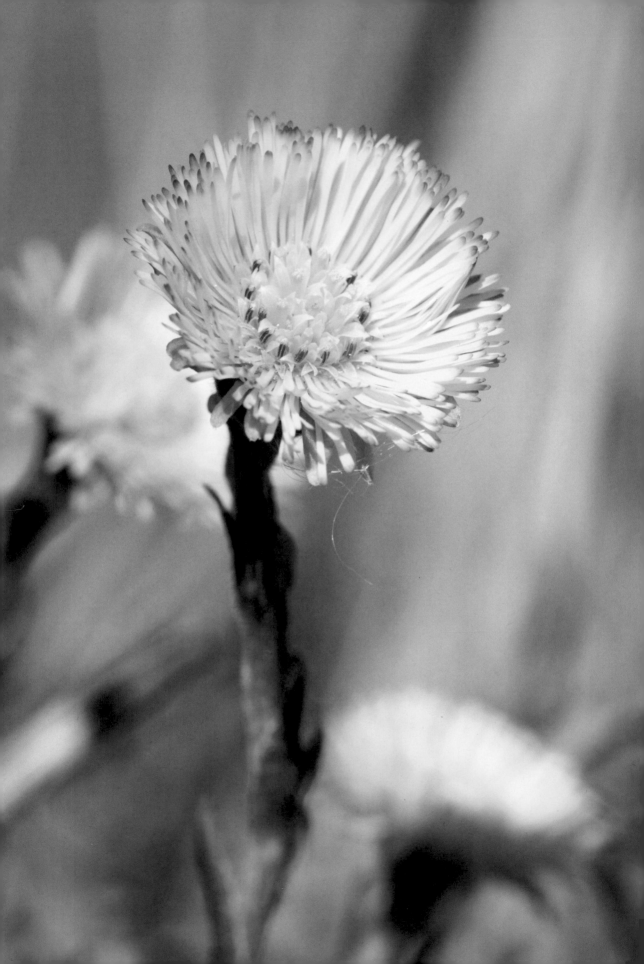

Coltsfoot
Tussilago farfara

Parts used: Leaves and flowers.

Properties/Actions: Antitussive, expectorant, demulcent, anti-inflammatory, astringent, antispasmodic.

Benefits: Traditional herb used for coughs and irritating respiratory issues including chronic emphysema and silicosis.

Can help immensely to recover after damage from smoking.

Suggested uses: Infusion, tincture.

Growing, harvesting, and wild crafting tips and specifics: Found wild commonly along roadsides, pathways, and the edges of forest and field. Leaf looks like a colt's foot! Small yellow dandelion-like flowers in the spring. Harvest leaves anytime, but they're best in fall when fully mature.

Cautions: Should not be used longer than 6 consecutive weeks per year, due to some alkaloids that may cause liver toxicity. Contraindicated while pregnant or nursing.

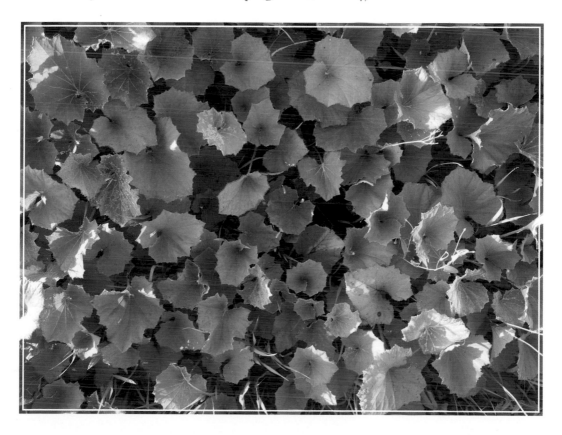

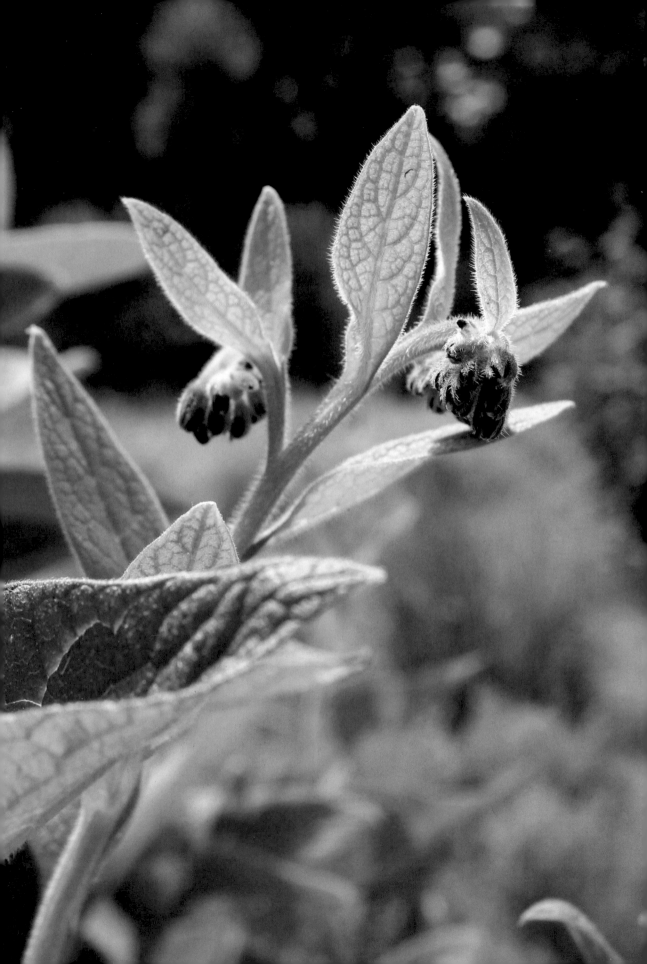

Comfrey
Symphytum officinale

Parts used: Leaves, roots.

Properties/Actions: Tonic, demulcent, expectorant, vulnerary, astringent.

Benefits: Rapidly promotes healing of wounds, sprains, bruises, burns, broken bones, sores, and ulcers. Has incredible results because it increases cell proliferation, both internally and externally.

Suggested uses: Infusion (leaf), decoction (root), herbal oil, salve, poultice, powder.

Growing, harvesting, and wild crafting tips and specifics: Perennial. Start from cuttings, or divided roots. Will take easily, and spread throughout the garden a lot, if not kept contained. If needed, keep contained by planting in a container, or weeding it out from unwanted locations.

Cautions: Comfrey has been used internally for thousands of years but just recently has become controversial due to a study concerning certain pyrilizidine alkaloids that it contains that can cause liver dysfunction. This study was done by feeding the roots to rats, who then developed tumors. This has never translated directly to humans, and, above ground, this plant does not contain high levels of this alkaloid.

The healing of wounds can be so rapid with the use of comfrey topically, that it is important to make sure the wound is very clean before applying comfrey, so that it does not lock in any kind of unfriendly bacteria, causing a trapped infection.

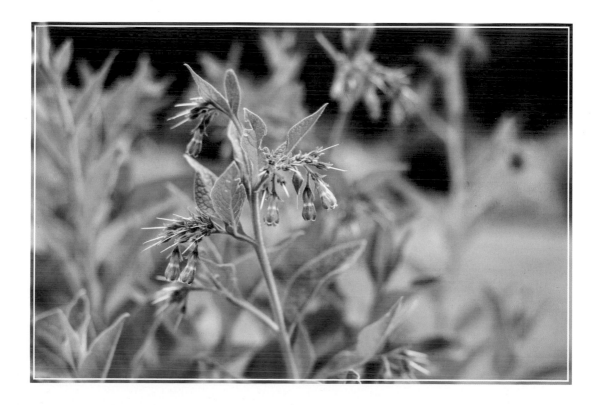

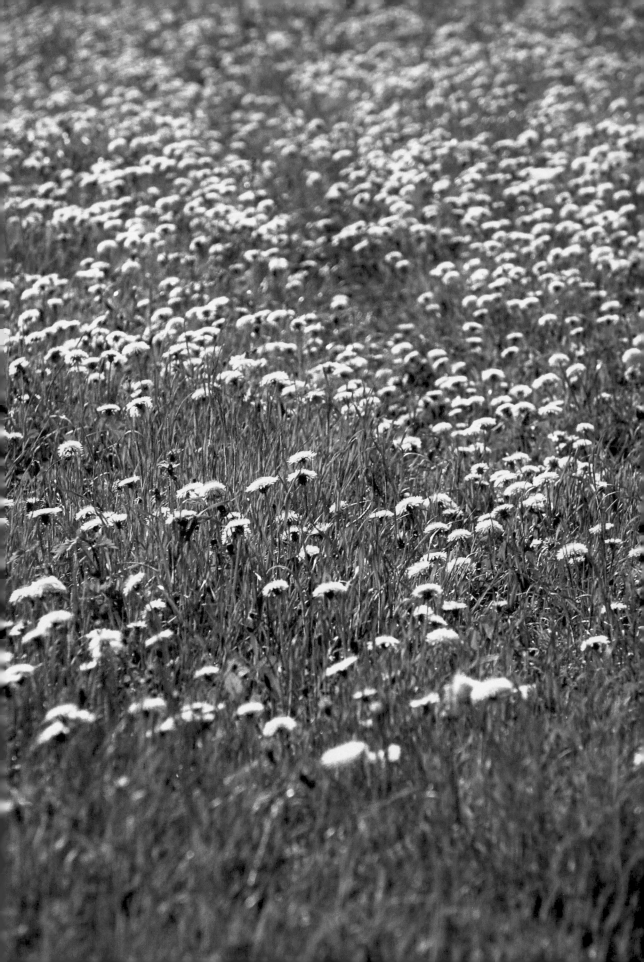

Dandelion
Taraxacum officinale

Parts used: Whole plant, leaves, flowers, roots.

Properties/Actions: Diuretic, stomachic, cholagogue, choleretic, alterative, tonic.

Benefits: Beneficial for liver problems, urinary tract infections, skin eruptions, high blood pressure, arthritis, gout, irregular blood sugar levels, skin diseases, women's imbalances, indigestion (due to bitter quality).

Helpful with weight loss and water retention due to high diuretic effect.

When root is roasted, makes a nice coffee substitute beverage.

Suggested uses: Infusion, decoction, tincture, capsule, wine.

Growing, harvesting, and wild crafting tips and specifics: Biennial. They spread prolifically as seeds are scattered by the wind. Dandelions are one of the most common "weeds." They are incredibly tenacious, even when sprayed many times with chemicals, they often survive. Will grow in the smallest cracks in sidewalks, and in the poorest soil. They bloom in the day and close at night.

The young leaves are best for eating. The flowers and leaves, right at the time of blooming, are great for tea or tincture, and the second-year roots have more potency to be tinctured or decocted.

Cautions: Contraindicated in bile duct obstruction and acute gall bladder inflammation.

I, doctor dandelion, affect ze liver most profoundly, encouraging its juices, strengthening and nourishing its ability to help you live. I help you function better, eh? I make you strong, and sure of yourself. You leave it to doctor dandelion. I improve your breasts, and your stomach, and even your guts, eh? I get rid of stuff in ze way, no matter what: any kind of blockage, resistance, doubt. And if you need, I put you to sleep. For the hard jobs, you get burdock to work with me, eh? We all have a good time, chere!

—Susun Weed, *Healing Wise*

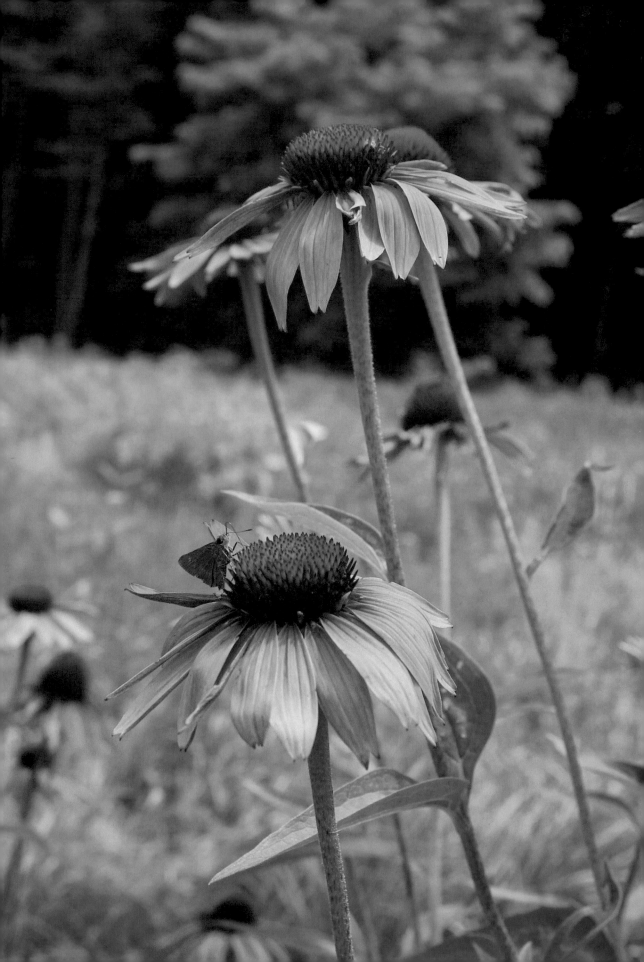

Echinacea
Echinacea purpurea and *angustifolia*

Parts used: Roots, flowers, and leaves.

Properties/Actions: Antimicrobial, anti-inflammatory, antiviral, antibacterial, antifungal.

Benefits: Eases colds and flus, fevers, lymphatic congestion, excessive coldnesss, dizziness, mental confusion, boils, skin eruptions, sores, infections, viruses.

All inflammatory conditions can be treated with echinacea.

Important to take in frequent small doses for ideal effectiveness.

Suggested uses: Infusion, decoction, tincture.

Growing, harvesting, and wild crafting tips and specifics: Perennial. Start from seed, or root division. Echinacea will grow well in most conditions, with the exceptions of very dry or very soggy soil.

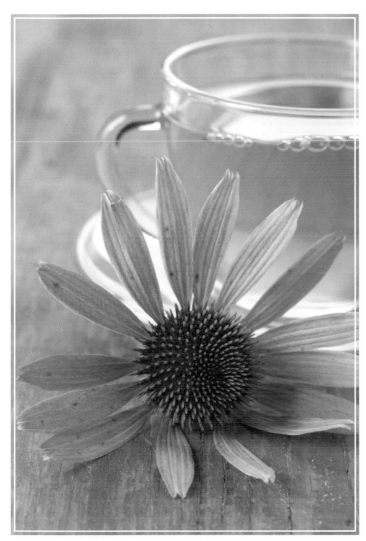

Cautions: Many herbalists believe that echinacea loses its effects if taken long term—more than 3–4 weeks at a time. May be wise to take a break after that time period, for about 2 weeks, and then start back up if need be.

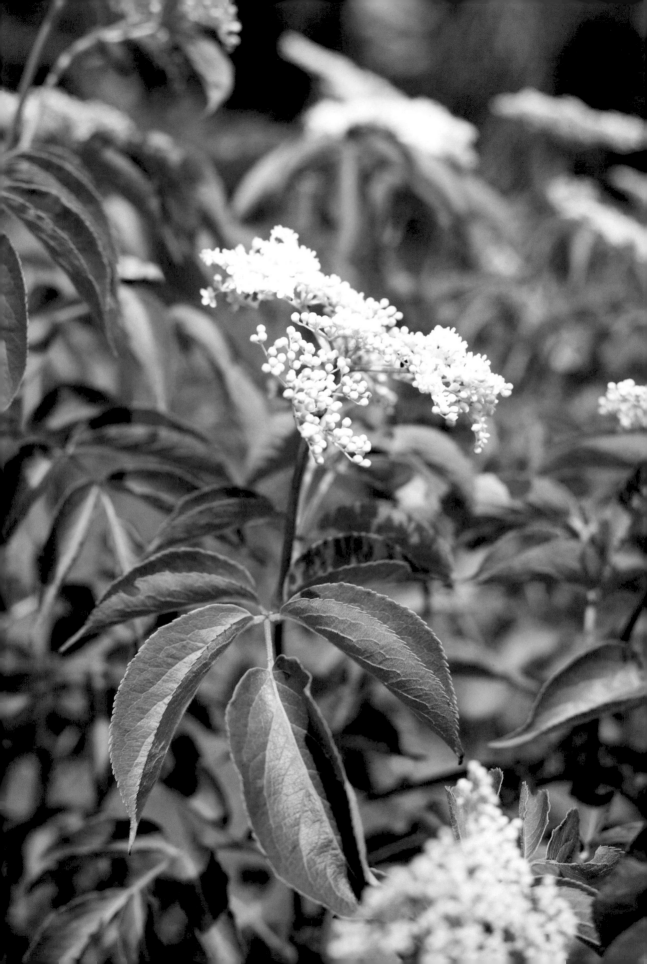

Elder
Sambucus nigra

Parts used: Flowers and berries.

Properties/Actions: Diaphoretic, alterative, stimulant, antirheumatic, antiviral.

Benefits: Eases colds, flus, fevers, acne, burns, rashes, wrinkles.

Suggested uses: Syrup (berries), infusion (flowers), herbal oil (flowers), salve (flowers).

Growing, harvesting, and wild crafting tips and specifics: Perennial. Divided roots. Prefers moist, well-drained, fertile soil.

Cautions: Only the black elderberry (nigra) is safe to use. The red variety is toxic.

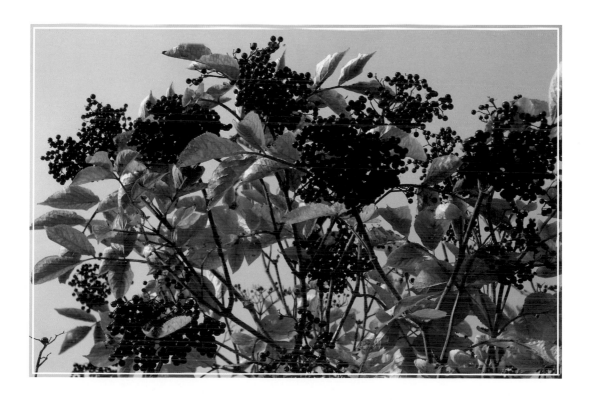

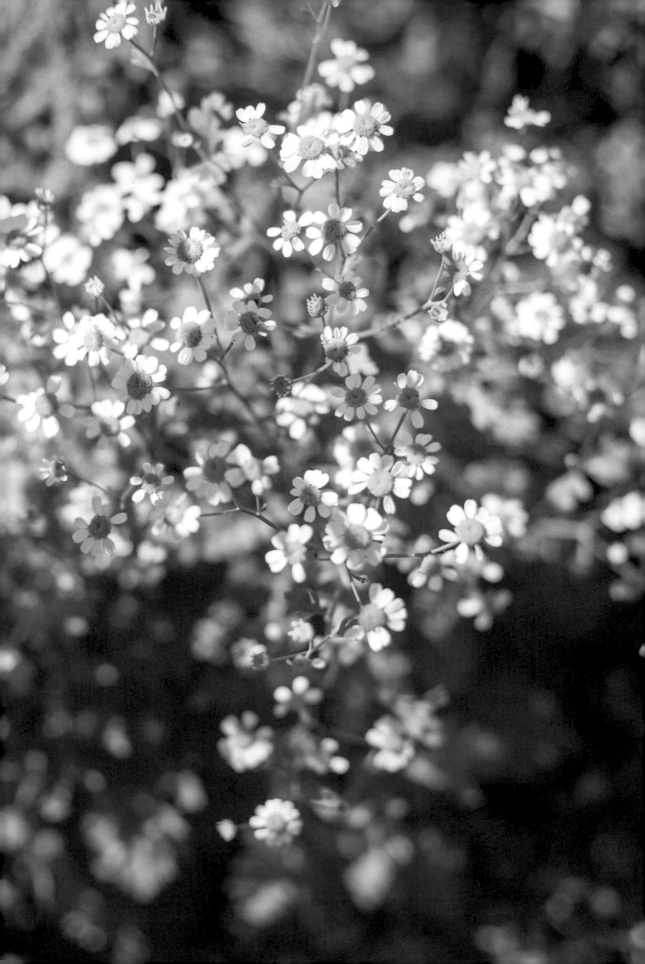

Feverfew
Tanacetum parthenium

Parts used: Flowering herb

Properties/Actions: Diaphoretic, anti-inflammatory.

Benefits: Used to equalize blood flow, effective in treating headaches and migraine, arthritis, colds and flu.

Suggested Use: Infusion, tincture, capsule.

Growing, harvesting, and wild crafting tips and specifics: Plant from seeds, seedlings, or root divisions, either in fall before danger of frost or in spring after the threat of frost has passed. It will self-sow throughout the garden. Likes dry, hot, sun. Needs very little attention in general.

Cautions: May cause ulceration of the mucous membranes when taken long-term. Best to take two-week breaks every few months if taking it regularly as a preventative.

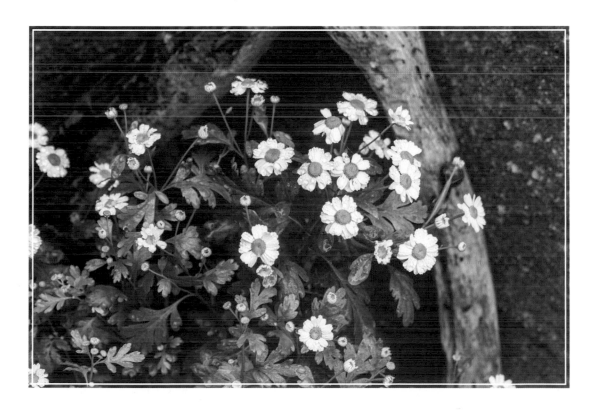

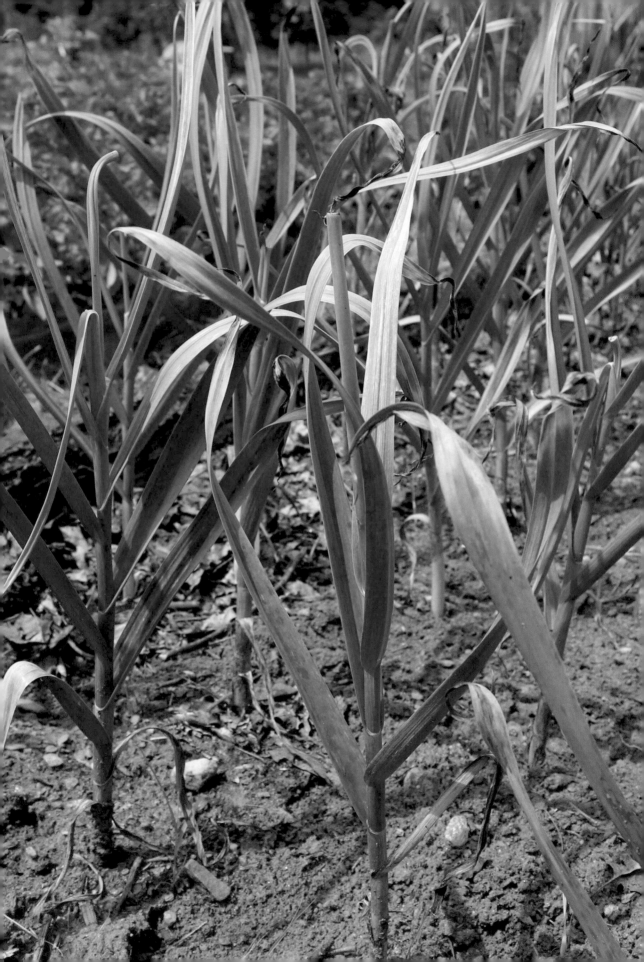

Garlic
Allium sativum

Parts used: Cloves.

Properties/Actions: Antibacterial, antifungal, antiparasitic, carminative, anticoagulant, antispasmodic, diaphoretic, hypotensive, cholagogue.

Benefits: Stimulates digestion and cardiovascular circulation. Eases colds and flus, hypertension, arthritic pain, candida.

Suggested uses: Tincture, powder (capsules), and most commonly, as food! Cooked or raw. See the recipe for Spicy Immunity Vinegar Tincture in the Simple Home Remedies section!

Growing, harvesting, and wild crafting tips and specifics: Annual. Plant in fall, late October or early November. Likes rich, well-drained soil, neutral pH.

To plant: Separate the cloves from a bulb of garlic from the last year. Each clove will grow its own bulb for next year! Make sure the cloves you are planting are nicely formed and in good condition, and are covered completely with at least a layer of skin. Plant about 4 inches down in the soil, 6 inches apart. Mulch well for the winter. In the spring after the danger of frost has passed, clear away the mulch, and the young garlic shoots will begin to poke through. The garlic will be ready to harvest around late July, once the aboveground parts have turned at least ¾ yellow/brown.

Pull from the ground, clean off excess soil, and hang to dry (cure) in a well-ventilated, shady, cool place such as a barn, shed, mudroom, or basement.

Fresh garlic is great to eat and use as well as cured garlic. Once it is cured, it will last the year if stored in a cool dry place. You can cut off the stalks once it's cured.

Cautions: Contraindicated for those who suffer from insomnia, dehydration, impending surgery, or acute inflammation.

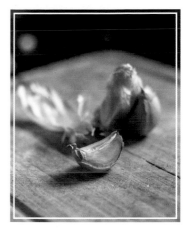

Garlic, a well-known culinary herb, is thought to have originated in the high plains of west central Asia and has been used medicinally for some five thousand years. This is the most powerful herb for the treatment of antibiotic-resistant disease. No other herb comes close to the multiple system actions of garlic, its antibiotic activity, and its immune-potentiating power.

—Stephen Harrod Buhner,
Herbal Antibiotics;
Natural Alternatives for
Treating
Drug-Resistant Bacteria

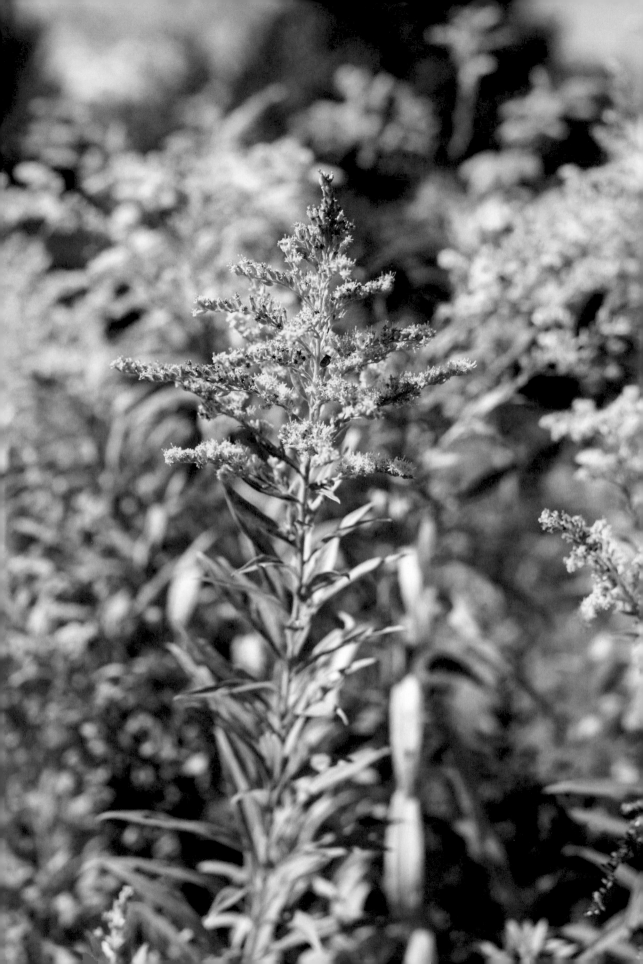

Goldenrod
Solidago Canadensis

Parts used: Leaves, stems, flowers

Properties/Actions: Anti-fungal, diuretic, diaphoretic, anti-inflammatory, expectorant, astringent, carminative.

Benefits: Strengthens and tones the bladder, urinary tract, and kidneys. Used for wounds and burns, as well as sore muscles and arthritis pain.

Suggested uses: Infusion, tincture, oil, poultice, powder.

Growing, harvesting, and wild crafting tips and specifics: Gather leaves, stems, and flowers just as the flowers are opening, or right before. Harvest in late summer to early fall. Grows prolifically in fields and edges.

Cautions: None known.

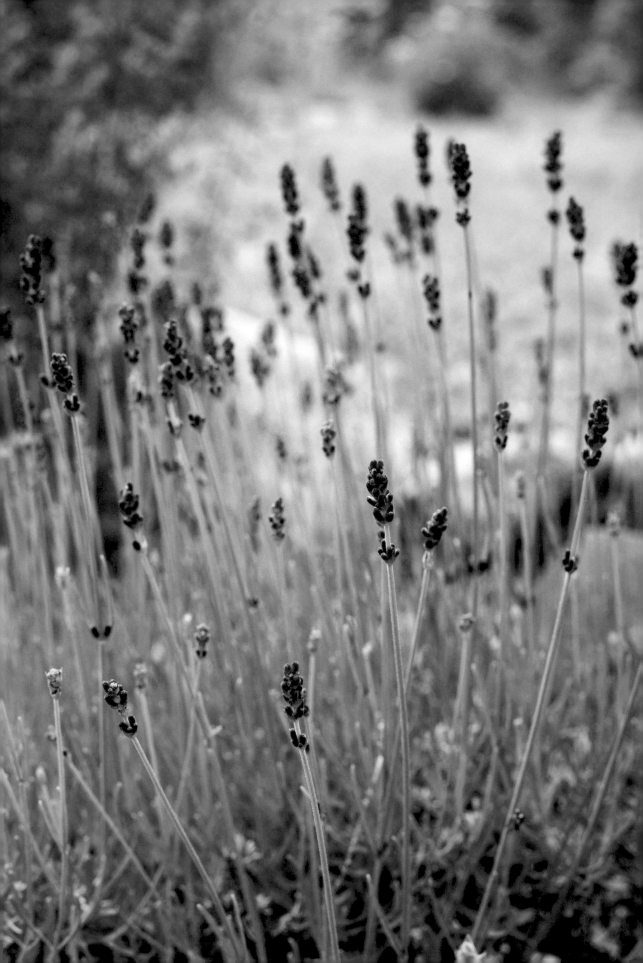

Lavender
Lavendula angustifolia, L. officinalis

Parts used: Flowers

Properties/Actions: Aromatic, carminative, antispasmodic, antidepressant.

Benefits: Great for emotional upset and calming the nervous system, soothing through aromatherapy use (such as essential oil in a bath or a diffuser). Used widely in body care products and to prevent insect bites and wool-eating moths in drawers. Essential oil can be used as topical first aid for soothing burns.

Suggested uses: Infusion, tincture, bath, lotion, insect repellent, salve/oil.

Growing, harvesting, and wild crafting tips and specifics: Perennial. Prefers lots of sun and dry weather. Sandy soil. Plant from divided roots, either in fall before danger of frost or in spring after the threat of frost has passed. Mulch well to ensure overwintering.

Cautions: Contraindicated in pregnancy (internally) due to emmenagogue effects unless used under the guidance of an herbalist.

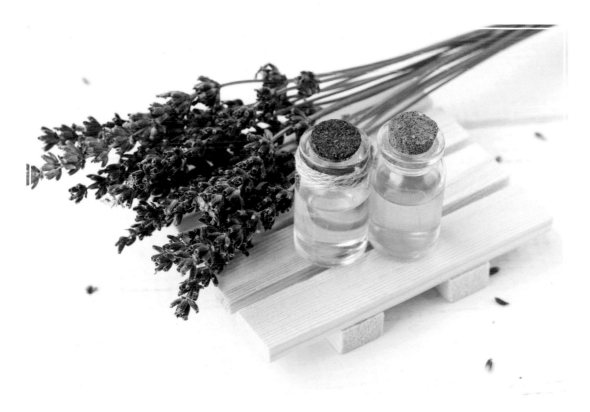

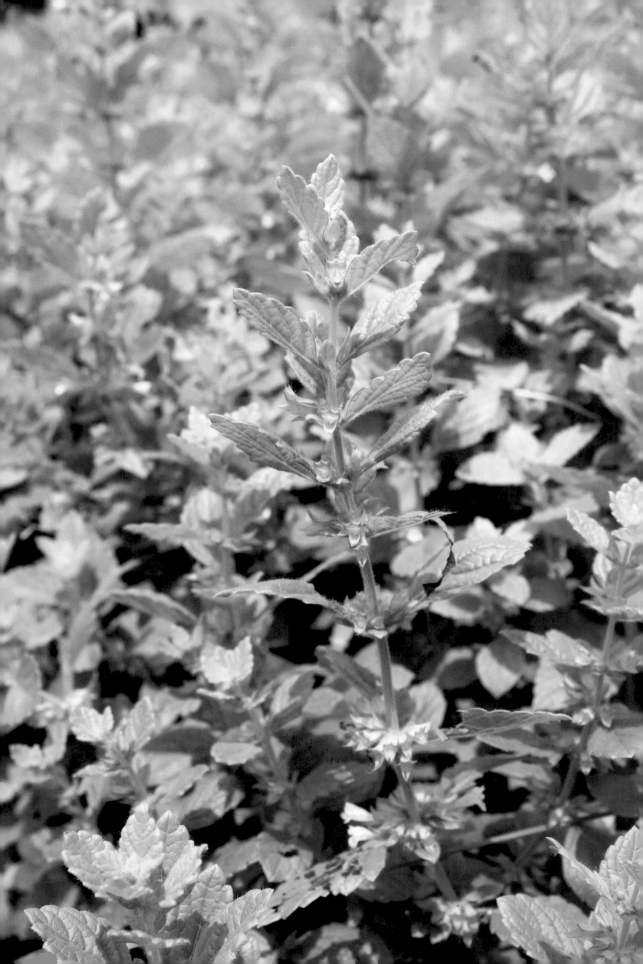

Lemon Balm
Melissa officinalis

Parts used: Leaves.

Properties/Actions: Diaphoretic, calmative, stomachic, carminative, antispasmodic, emmenagogue, nervine, sedative, antiviral, antidepressant.

Benefits: Eases digestive problems, nervousness, insomnia, depression, migraines, stress, hypertension, herpes symplex and zoster, restlessness, palpitations, fevers.

Very good for children, mild and pleasant tasting. Generally calms and soothes.

Suggested uses: Infusion, salve.

Growing, harvesting, and wild crafting tips and specifics: Perennial. Grows and spreads prolifically. It will pop up in random places around the garden! Divide roots, or start from seed indoors in late winter or early spring. Transplant into garden after danger of frost.

Can usually yield many harvests throughout the summer into the fall.

Best used fresh.

Cautions: Contraindicated with hypothyroidism.

When I was three years old, I got one chicken pock on my cheek. My mom brought me to the doctor to check in and see if this would be enough to give me immunity for life. The answer was unsure at that time, but I never got chicken pox again in childhood, so we thought the coast was clear.

Just around the time of my twenty-seventh birthday, I was exposed to chicken pox through one of my nieces, and about two weeks later I started to have a few itchy spots on my scalp. I did not suspect chicken pox (herpes zoster) one bit, but wondered what it could be, thinking dry skin, bug bites, maybe lice?! A few more days went by, and I woke up one morning absolutely *covered*, from head to toe in pox! Not only was the sight of myself incredibly startling, but I itched in pain—not an itch you can scratch—and I was sick with fever.

Getting chicken pox as an adult is awful—it lasts longer and is more intense than in childhood. But I have to say, lemon balm really does help here. I drank a lot of lemon balm infusion over the course of the illness, and it helped shorten the length and ease the symptoms. Lemon balm is such a nice medicine for children, and luckily most people get chicken pox when they are young.

When it was all said and done and the pox were gone, I was grateful to have the immunity finally, and felt stronger for it. But then I knew that now I could get shingles (same herpes zoster virus that only people who've had pox can get). Sure enough, a few years later, when I was about eight months pregnant with my first child, I got shingles! It manifested on a nerve pathway right on the bottom of my big pregnant belly and was painful and troubling indeed. Again, lemon balm came to my aid. The severe pain only lasted a few days, and there was no transmission to the baby. All was fine in the end. And no sign of this virus since!

—Alyssa

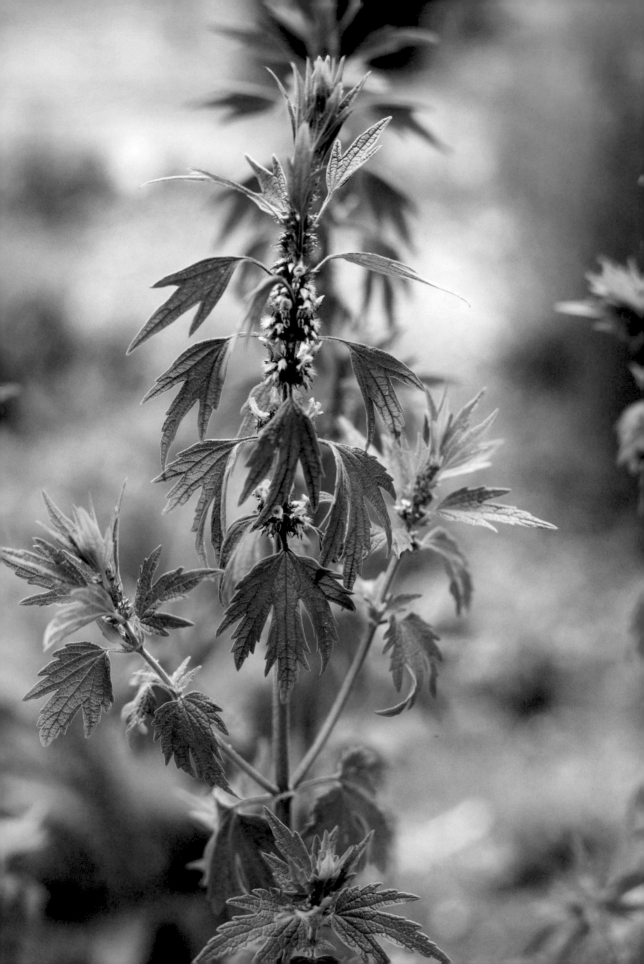

Motherwort
Leonurus cardiaca

Parts used: Leaves, stems, flower (in bud stage).

Properties/Actions: Emmenagogue, antispasmodic, nervine, diuretic, carminative, female tonic.

Benefits: Strengthens the heart (emotionally and physically), beneficial for nerve pain, high blood pressure, nervous palpitation, disturbed sleep, general pain relief, emotional turbulence, hysteria, convulsions.

Can be greatly beneficial for labor pains, after birth pains, and restoration of spirit and body after the birth of a baby.

Suggested uses: Tincture, infusion.

Growing, harvesting, and wild crafting tips and specifics: Perennial. Found wild along stream beds. Very forgiving and flexible in most growing and soil conditions. Will self-seed prolifically if the seed is allowed to mature and spread. Start from seed after freezing them for several months or plant seeds in the ground in the fall, so the winter season naturally stratifies (freezes) them. Also can be started by root division.

Cautions: Avoid during pregnancy. Some say it has addicting qualities when used long term for depression/anxiety/stress. Best to take breaks now and then, if taking it regularly.

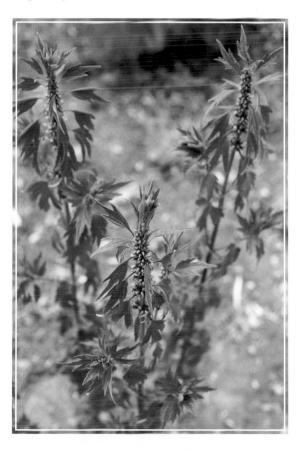

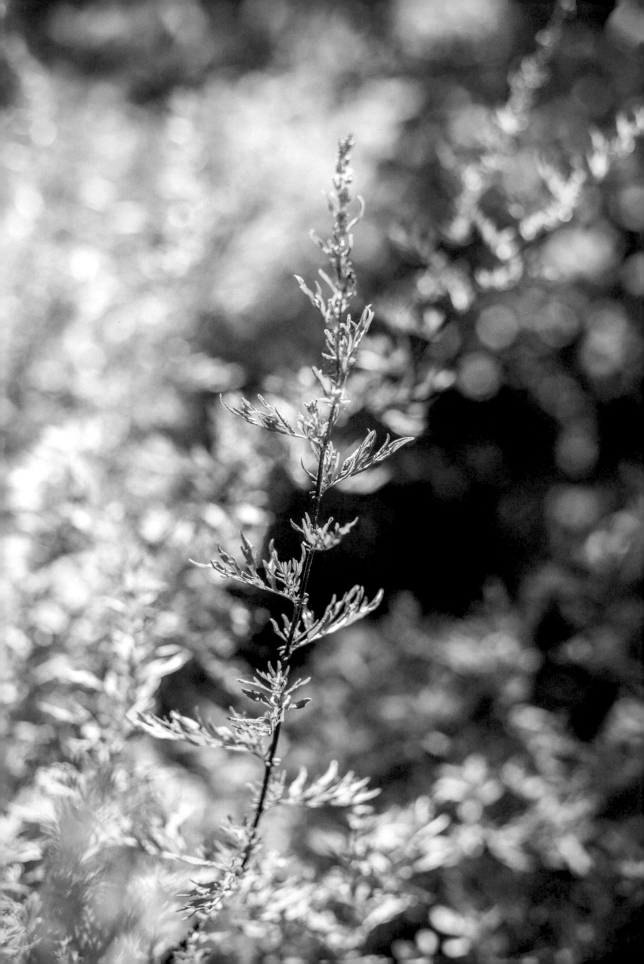

Mugwort
Artemisia vulgaris

Parts used: Leaves

Properties/Actions: Cholagogue, vermifuge, emmenagogue, hemostatic, antispasmodic, diaphoretic, mild narcotic, bitter tonic.

Benefits: Helps with nervousness. Calms uncontrollable shaking, liver problems, stomach issues. Used in ritual purification. Helps to correct suppressed menstruation, insomnia.

Suggested uses: Infusion, tincture, smudge.

Growing, harvesting, and wild crafting tips and specifics: Perennial. Super easy to grow, mugwort self-seeds, spreads, and gets quite tall. Harvest in late summer through fall. Plant from seed or from divided roots, either in fall before danger of frost or in spring after the threat of frost has passed. Great plant for beginner gardeners. Also found wild, mostly along roadsides and field edges.

Cautions: People who have allergies to plants in the wormwood family may get rash from mugwort.

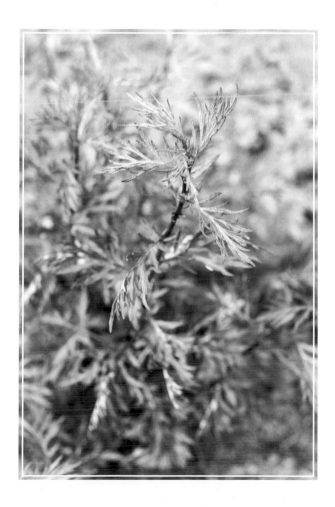

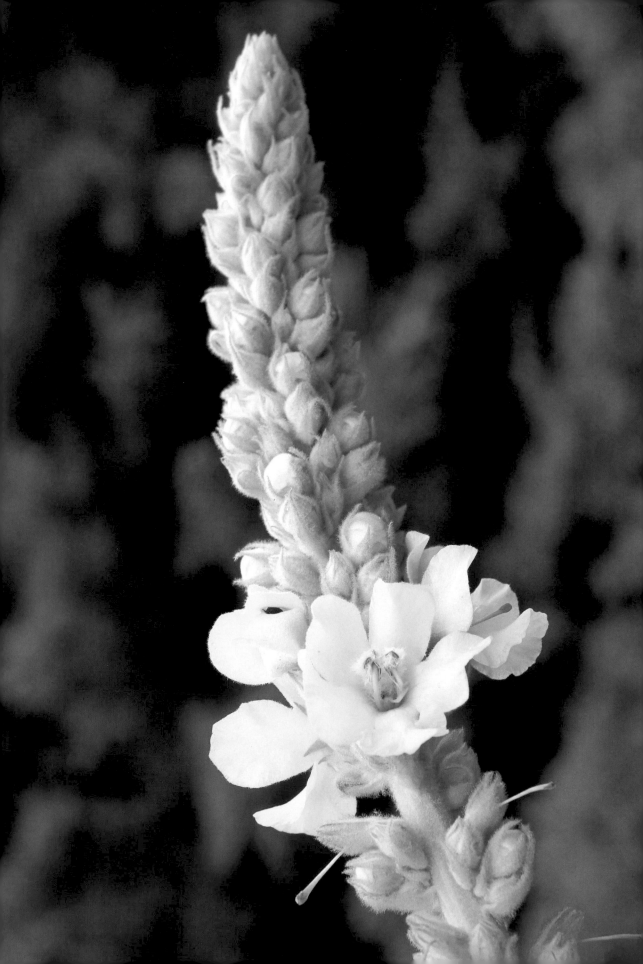

Mullein
Verbascum thapsus

Parts used: Leaf, flower, root.

Properties/Actions: Expectorant, demulcent, anodyne, vulnerary, antitussive, alterative, astringent.

Benefits: Eases hoarseness, coughs, bronchitis, whooping cough, asthma, hay fever.

Colic, constipation, facial neuralgia, and urinary tract infections.

Externally, the flowers infused into oil are used for earaches/infections—often along with garlic and/or thyme.

Suggested uses: Infusion, tincture, herbal oil (flowers).

Growing, harvesting, and wild crafting tips and specifics: Biennial. Mullein is what we call a "pioneer" plant, meaning it will be one of the first plants to grow in a disturbed area, whether from fire or logging, etc. It grows well in poor soil, but prefers sunny spots.

Cautions: None available at this time.

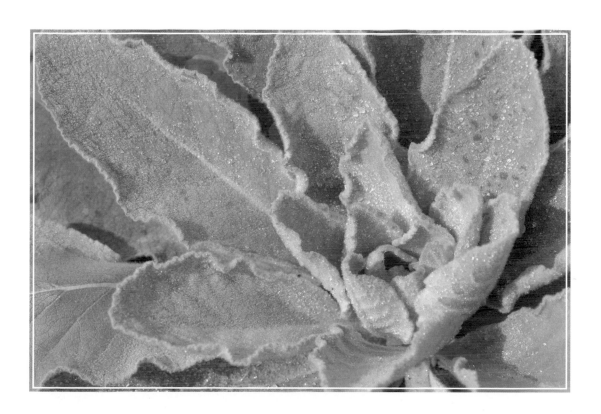

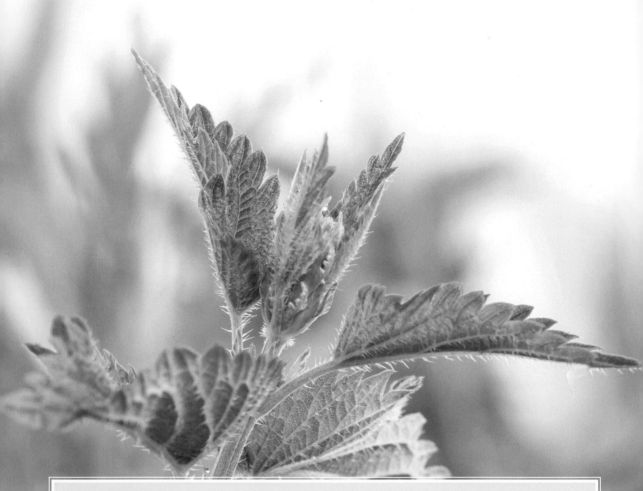

Ode to Nettle

It would be difficult to do, because I have such deep love for so many herbs, but, if I had to pick a favorite that I hold dearest to my heart . . . it would be nettle.

Nettle has been such a faithful and steadfast daily herbal ally for me for about ten years. I feel that we have merged and become one, that when I drink nettle infusion, it is bonding with my very blood, and every cell of my body. I sometimes feel like Popeye when I drink my infusion, strong and robust. I incorporate it into most all of my blends, but mostly I love to drink it straight, and strong. I usually brew up a quart and let it stand overnight, excited to unveil my deep green drink in the morning. It feels so nourishing and hydrating—similar to an electrolyte drink such as fresh coconut water.

Nettle has been especially beneficial for me during my two pregnancies. I drank it almost every day, sometimes alternating with red raspberry leaf, and a few others, but for the most part nettle was my drink of choice. I felt that it helped me with all aspects and symptoms of pregnancy making for a healthy, enjoyable time in my life. I also believe that it delivered vitamin K to my infants, which they so need for proper blood clotting in the beginning weeks of life.

I feel a foundation of health and strength in my body, which I attribute in large part to the regular consumption of nettle. I rarely drink plain water—it does not feel as hydrating!

When my husband and I found the land we wanted to buy and build our home on, along with some other family members, we had to name our new road. I really tried to convince everyone that Nettle Hill was the way to go! Alas, images and feelings of stinginess arose for everyone, and we ended up going with Harvest Hill.

To me, when I come across nettle in the wild, or as a weed that snuck into my garden, it's exciting! Lively! It represents deep radiant health.

—Alyssa

Nettle
Urtica urens

Parts used: Leaves, sometimes roots.

Properties/Actions: Tonic, astringent, diuretic, hemostatic, galactagogue, nutritive, expectorant.

Benefits: Nettles are a tonic that will benefit the whole body taken over long periods of time. Nettles are filled with minerals, vitamins, and chlorophyll. Especially ideal in treating anemia. Drinking infusion of nettle is useful for asthma, urinary complaints, kidney stones, and overall kidney health; helpful for cystitis, diarrhea, hemorrhoids, and chronic arthritic and rheumatic problems.

Topically, powdered nettles can be put directly onto a bleeding wound to stop bleeding. A brief application of fresh leaves brushed directly onto an arthritic area will provide some relief through release of histamine (see cautions below).

Nettles nourish the scalp to promote hair health and growth.

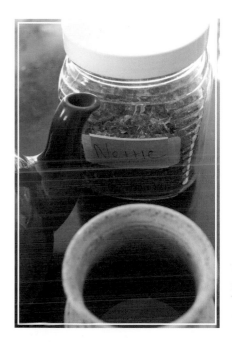

Suggested uses: Infusion, tincture, powder directly on wounds, infused into apple cider vinegar as hair tonic, eaten in soups, breads, or salads. Once they are dried or cooked, the sting is gone.

Growing, harvesting, and wild crafting tips and specifics: Nettles are found in the wild, usually in farm fields where manure has been, or on the forest edges. The best time to collect the leaves is when they are fresh spring shoots, around April to May. The younger they are the more filled with vital nutrients, and the less likely to sting. Wearing gloves to harvest is recommended unless you have arthritic hands and/or like the feeling of the light stinging sensation. Likes nitrogen rich soil, wetter conditions, and sun to mostly shade.

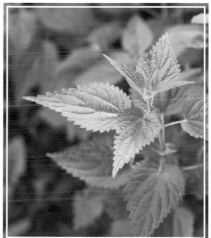

Cautions: The sting! Though not harmful, it lingers quite a while and can be really uncomfortable for some people, and may cause a mild to severe rash. The rash can be treated by rubbing plantain leaves or yellow dock leaves directly onto the effected area, which are usually found growing right nearby.

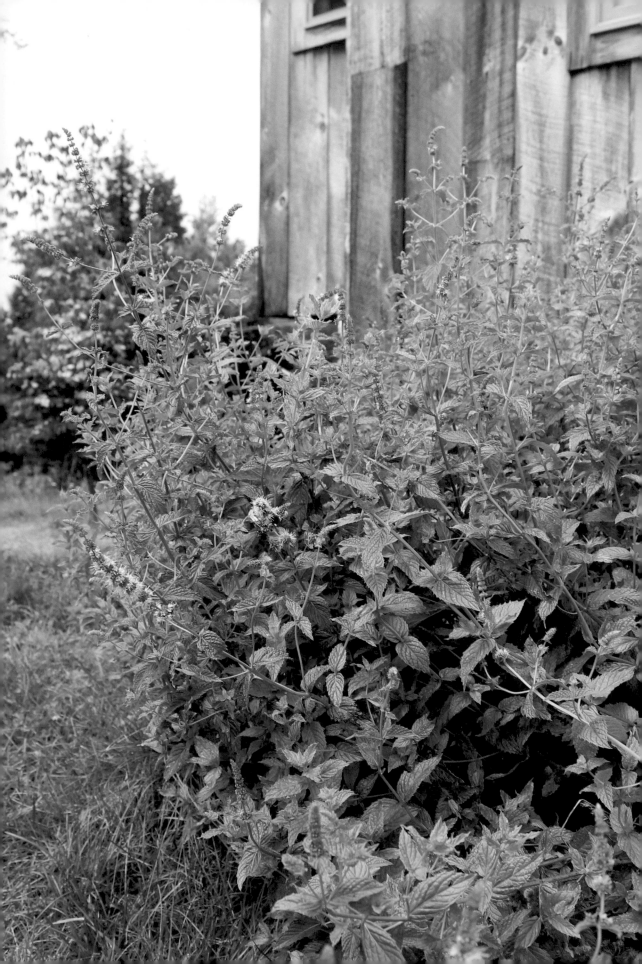

Peppermint
Mentha piperita

Parts used: Leaves.

Properties/Actions: Antispasmodic, carminative, diaphoretic, analgesic (externally), stimulant, disinfectant, choleretic, cholagogue.

Benefits: Eases general indigestion, flatulence, colic, irritable bowel syndrome, nausea, vomiting, cold and flu, stings and bites, itchy skin.

Suggested uses: Infusion, essential oil (for topical uses such as bites, stings, itchy skin).

Growing, harvesting, and wild crafting tips and specifics: Perennial. Spreads easily. prefers moist, rich soil. Start from seed or root division.

Best to keep in a container or contained garden bed to prevent it from taking over your whole garden.

Cautions: Contraindicated in high quantities during pregnancy due to emmenagogue effect.

Around thirty years ago I met a woman who was born in Germany in the late 1800s. She was in her herb garden in Western Massachusetts, and I was a "back-to-the-lander" (child born in the 1960s) and interested in growing my own herbs. Irma was around ninety-five years old then, and still going strong. She had bright blue eyes and white hair held in a bun at the nape of her neck. She had one of those classic flowered aprons on as she bent over her wheelbarrow talking to herself in German. Since German was my minor as a comp-lit major, I of course approached her and asked her what she was growing. We began a nice conversation, which evolved into a discussion on growing herbs and the health benefits.

Irma told me that if I wanted to live to ninety-five, "just use herbs and drink tea." She was very direct about that, but of course she was out there exercising every day with her wheelbarrow, weeding, walking around, even in her nineties. Well, she is long gone, and I still remember her words of wisdom, and now I grow my own herbs here in southern Vermont I swear by using peppermint as a soothing tea to aid digestion, and I grow lavender to use as an aromatic and therapeutic flower essence for the bath.

I grow and buy and forage for other herbs, like ginger, but my favorite herb to aid digestion (as an expert spokeswoman on digestive disease, it is part of my research for my books) is peppermint. It helps for all kinds of digestive distress, such as irritable bowel syndrome, diverticultis, and heartburn, it even helps me when I have a headache. I grow my own peppermint and make a tea from the leaves. I let the tea steep for a long time (I use one of those tea balls), and I sweeten it with honey. In summer, I use the fresh-grown mint leaves in black or green iced tea (I make a "sun tea") to flavor it and make the glass look pretty. (I also use mint leaves in my homemade mojitos!) This time of year, I have taken my leaves inside and I hang them upside down to dry so I can have the fragrant herb smell in the middle of winter.

—Dede

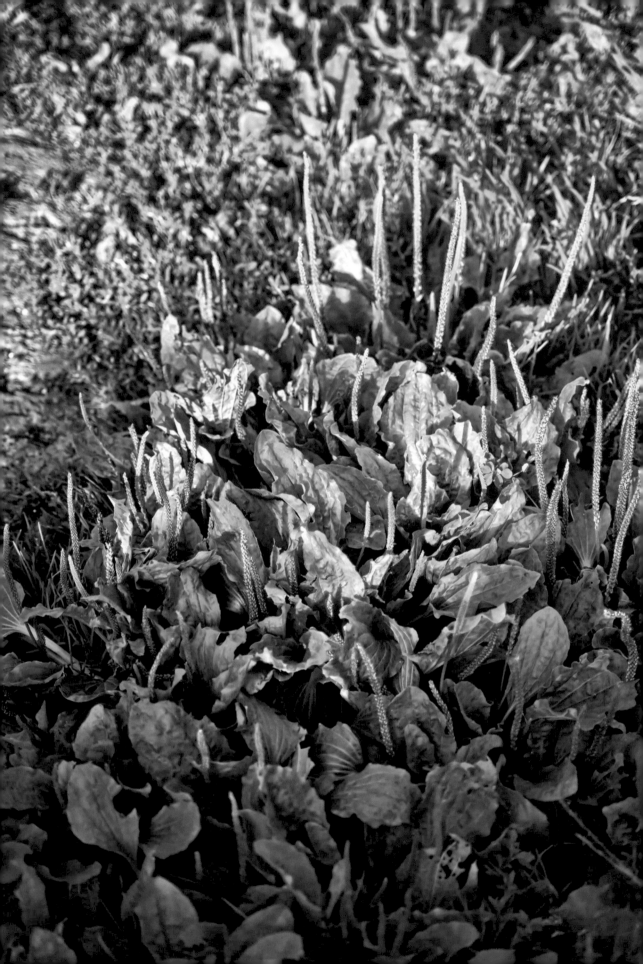

Plantain
Plantago species

Parts used: Leaves.

Properties/Actions: Diuretic, antiseptic, astringent, aperient, alterative, anti-inflammatory, mucilaginous.

Benefits: Taken internally, its demulcent action helps to heal urinary tract and respiratory infections. Also used internally for hepatitis and dysentery.

Topically, helps stop bleeding and promote healing of wounds. Effective first aid as a fresh poultice for stings, bites, cuts, and scrapes. It will also draw out splinters.

Suggested uses: Infusion, tincture, poultice with fresh masticated leaves or dry powder.

Growing, harvesting, and wild crafting tips and specifics: Perennial. Grows in any soil. Will thrive in sun or shade. There are over 200 varieties!

A very common "weed" in lawns and gardens and cracks in concrete.

Plantain was/is often called "White Man's Foot Print" by Native Americans, because it came from Europe, and quickly spread everywhere, all across the country.

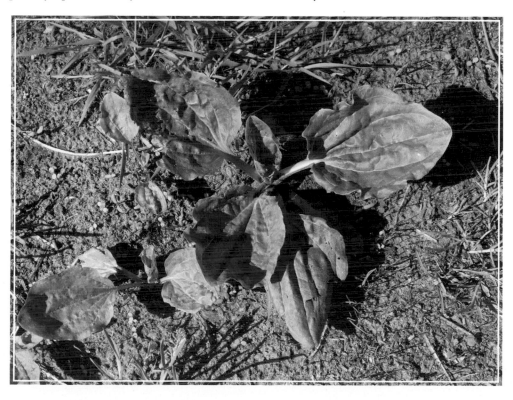

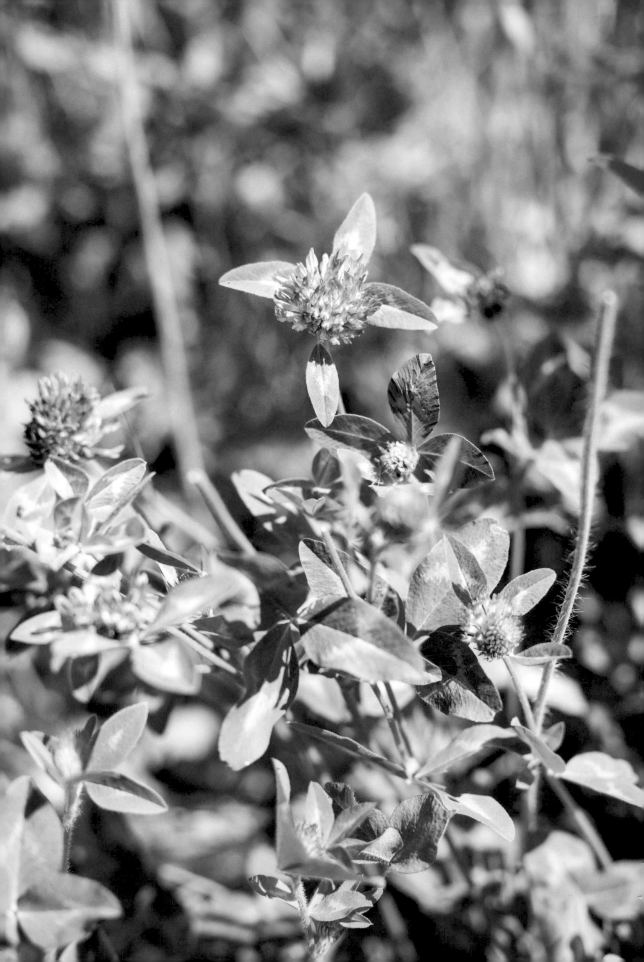

Red Clover

Trifolium pratense

Parts used: Flowers.

Properties/Actions: Alterative, antispasmodic, expectorant, sedative, antitumor.

Benefits: Eases skin complaints, coughs, colds, and any congestion.

Red clover is indicated for debilitated individuals, salivary gland congestion, and along with heat and massage can clear a stiff neck associated with swollen nodes.

Red clover is used for the treatment of cancer— usually combined in a formula with other herbs. Seek professional guidance here.

Suggested use: Infusion, tincture.

Growing, harvesting, and wild crafting tips and specifics: Perennial. Often found in fields/pastures. Prefers rich, fertile, well-drained soil. Flowers throughout the summer. Fun to harvest!

Cautions: Contraindicated in pregnancy and for individuals using blood-thinning drugs. Red clover is a blood thinner, so it can potentiate the effect of other blood-thinning substances.

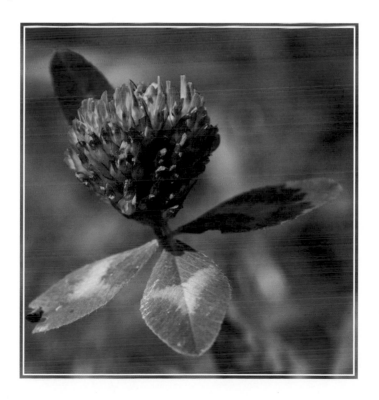

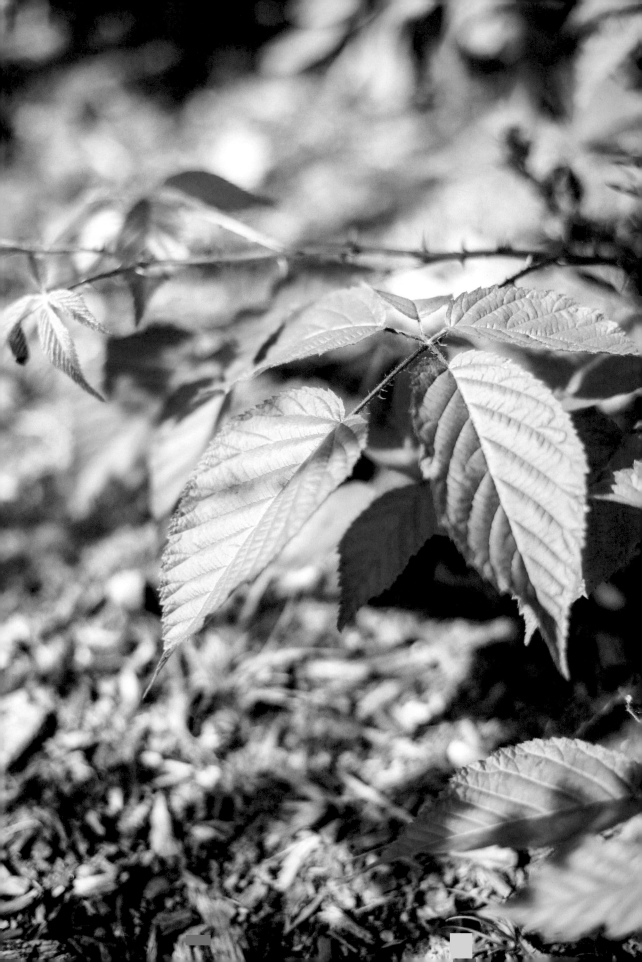

Red Raspberry
Rubus idaeus

Parts used: Leaf.

Properties/Actions: Astringent, uterine tonic, mild alterative, hemostatic.

Benefits: Take throughout pregnancy to tone and strengthen the uterus, help with delivery, give some iron and energy, and help prevent postpartum hemorrhage.

Effective for menstrual irregularity and cramps, and also reduces fevers.

High in minerals.

Suggested uses: Infusion, tincture.

Growing, harvesting, and wild crafting tips and specifics: Perennial. Grows in poor soil, in many conditions including sun and shade. Try and get young leaves when harvesting.

Cautions: Prickly! Wear gloves when harvesting.

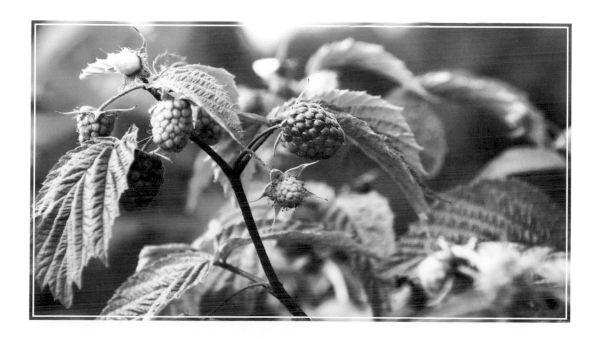

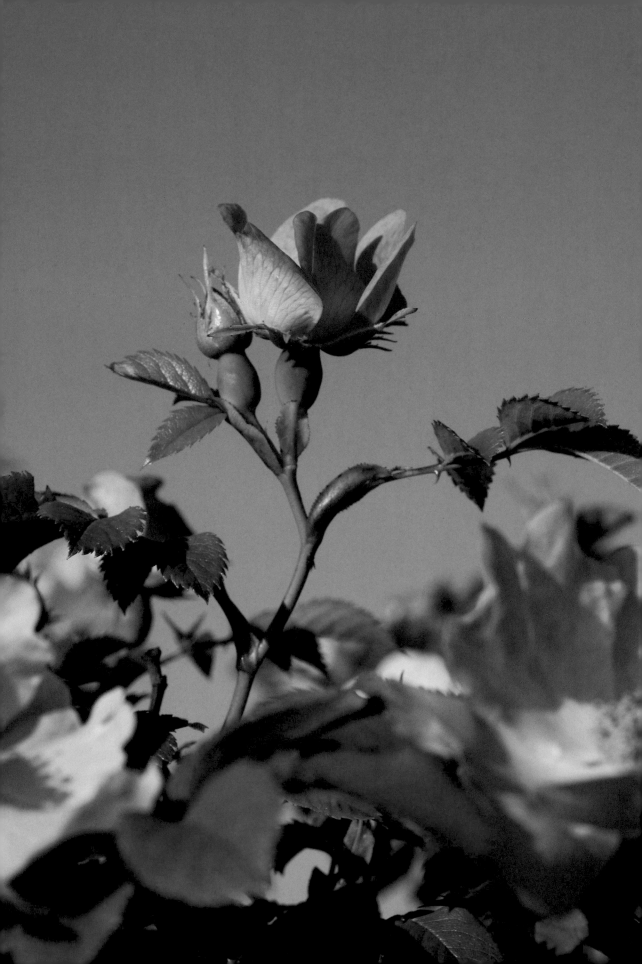

Rose (also called beach rose)
Rosa rugosa

Parts used: Petals and hips

Properties/Actions: Antidepressant, antispasmodic, aphrodisiac, astringent, antiviral, anti-inflammatory, blood tonic, digestive stimulant, kidney tonic, menstrual regulator.

Benefits: Colds, skin issues, headaches, stomach weakness, ease for heavy menstruation, sore throat, depression, insomnia.

Suggested uses: Infusion, tincture, lotion, salve, or added to a bath.

Growing, harvesting, and wild crafting tips and specifics: Grows wild along beaches and can be easily cultivated in temperate climates. Super prickly so use caution when harvesting. Wait until hips are red to harvest. Petals come in early summer, hips arrive mid to late summer. Prefer lots of sun and sandy soil.

Cautions: Use only rose species that are used for medicinal purposes (there are many in addition to *Rosa rugosa*)

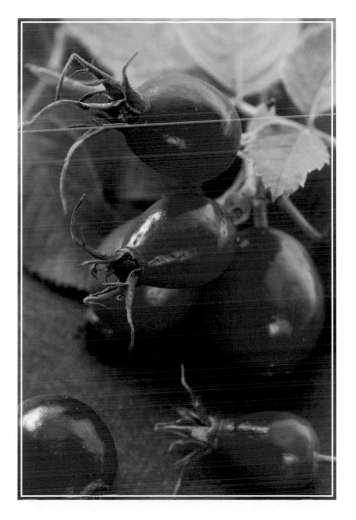

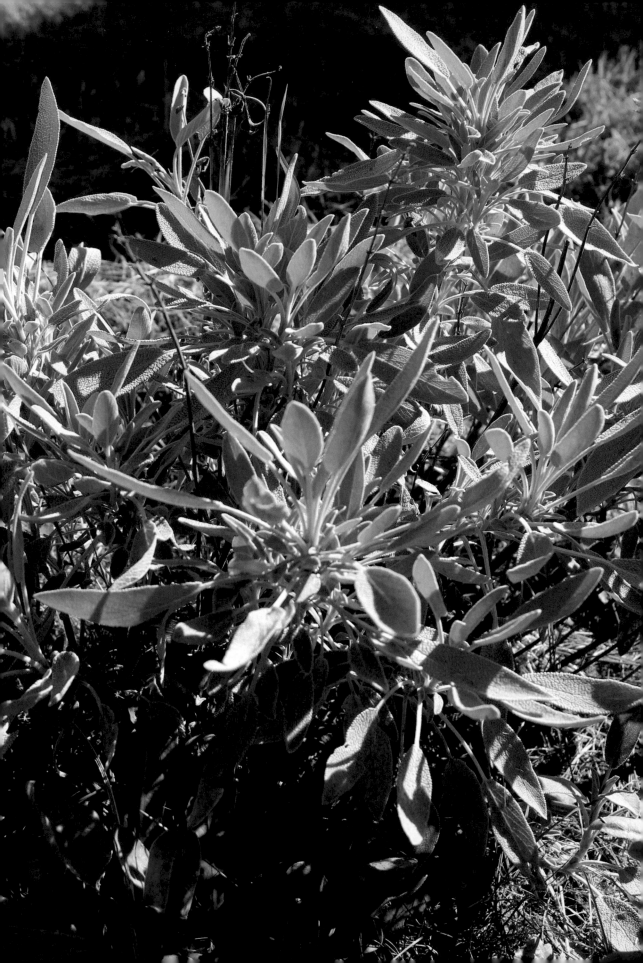

Sage
Salvia officinalis

Parts used: Leaves, whole above ground plant when flowers are in budding stage.

Properties/Actions: Diuretic, astringent, carminative, antibacterial.

Benefits: Reduces hot flashes/excessive perspiration, diarrhea, gas, burping, sore throats, cleansing and healing for gum ulcerations.

Can help with reduction of breast milk, which can be beneficial while weaning.

Suggested uses: Infusion, tincture, salve, poultice.

Growing, harvesting, and wild crafting tips and specifics: Perennial. Start from root divisions, seed, or cutting. If from seed, start indoors in late winter and transplant into the garden in spring.

Cautions: Contraindicated during pregnancy and breast feeding, due to abortifacient effect and reduced milk flow.

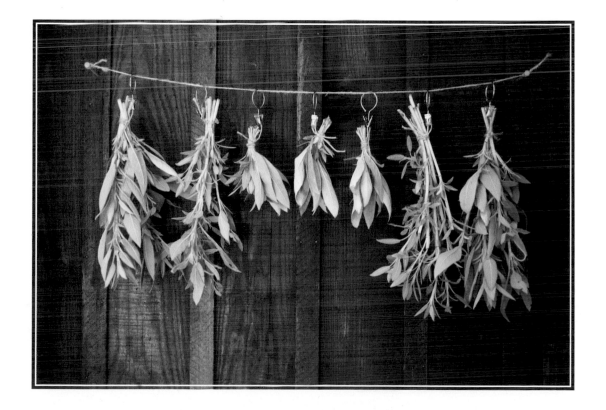

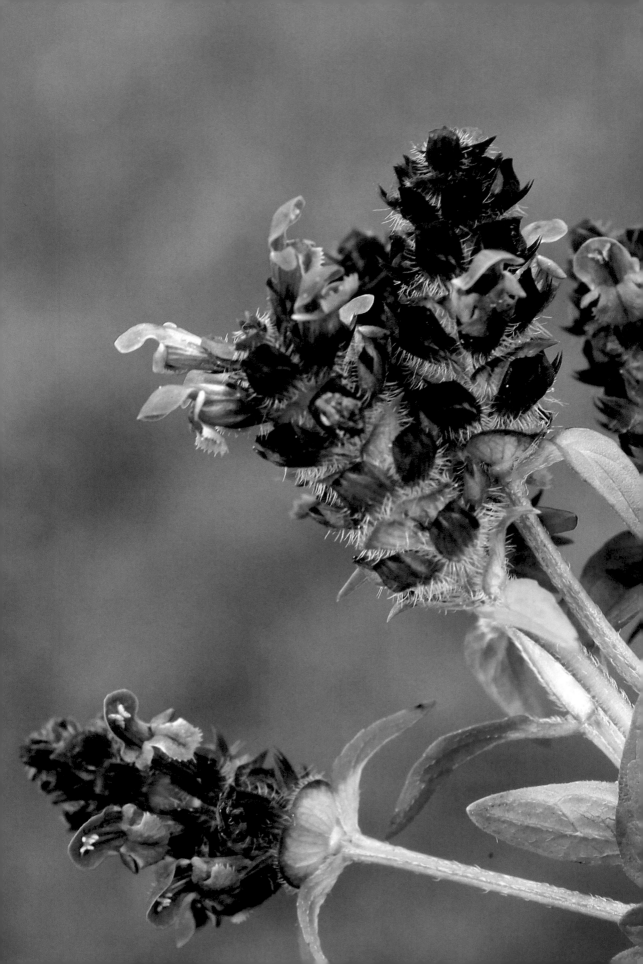

Self-heal
Prunella vulgaris

Parts used: Leaves and flowers.

Properties/Actions: Astringent, Anti-inflammatory, antipyretic, mild antiseptic, diuretic, detoxifier, hemostatic, vulnerary.

Benefits: Healing to cuts, wounds, and skin inflammations, boils. Is used to impede bleeding, and for sore throats and mouth ulcers. Useful lymphatic herb to help relieve fibrocystic breast tissue.

Suggested uses: Infusion, tincture, salve, gargle (using the infusion), poultice. Great in salads.

Growing, harvesting, and wild crafting tips and specifics: Perennial. Grows in pastures, along roadsides, and in wastelands. Will often pop up as a "weed" in your garden. Likes plenty of sun, but flexible with soil type.

Cautions: None at this time, very mild herb.

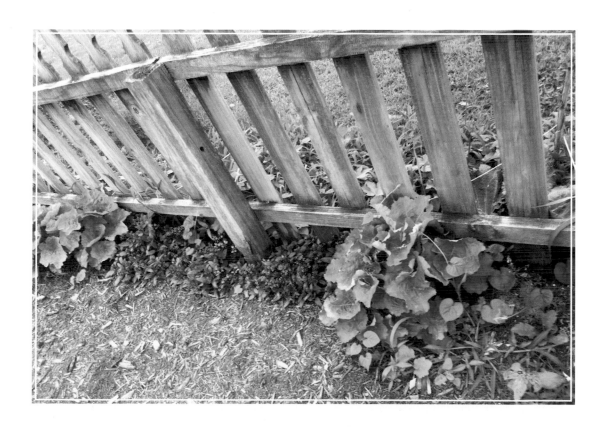

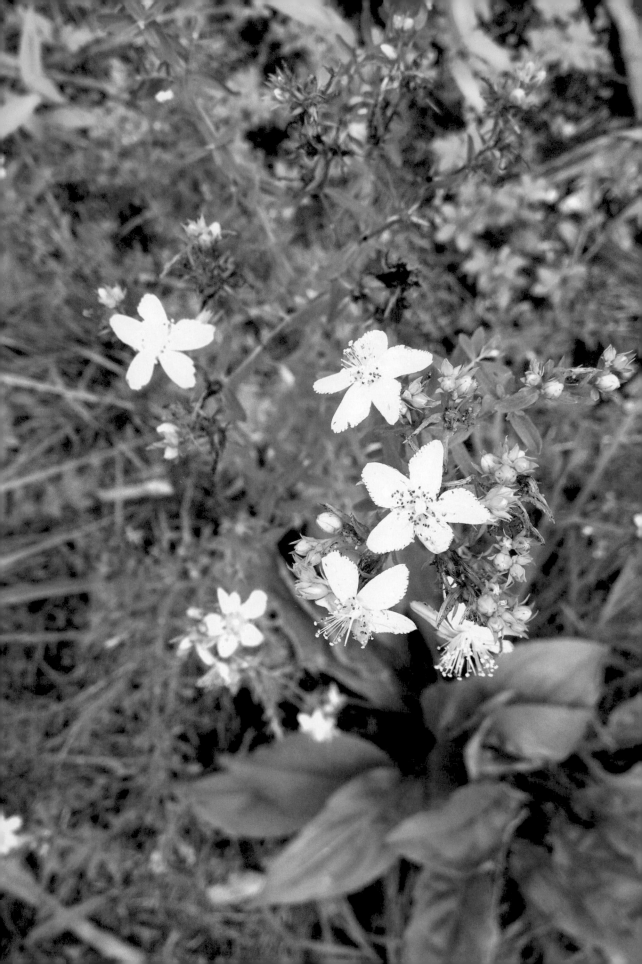

St. John's Wort
Hypericum perforatum

Parts used: Flowers, stem, leaves.

Properties/Actions: Anti-inflammatory, antidepressant, sedative, astringent, antiviral, nervine, antibacterial.

Benefits: Facilitates the body receiving sunlight, eases nervous exhaustion, nerve pain, depression, anxiety, feelings of being disconnected with the world, shingles, hemorrhoids, ulcers, muscular pain, diaper rash, and cradle cap.

Suggested uses: Tincture, infusion, capsule, herbal oil, salve.

Growing, harvesting, and wild crafting tips and specifics: Perennial. Blooms from June to August. Commonly found in dry gravelly soils, in pastures, and in mostly sunny locations.

Cautions: Contraindicated in pregnancy. May increase photosensitivity in fair-skinned people.

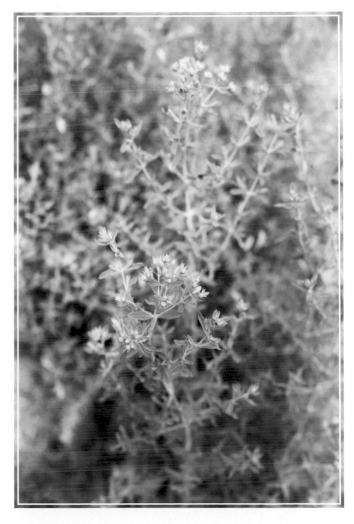

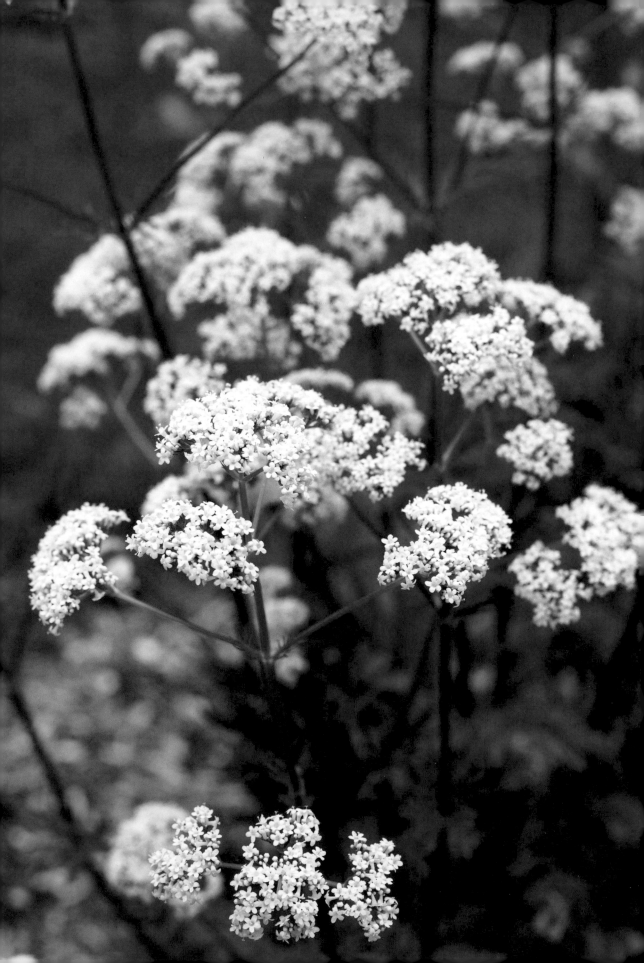

Valerian
Valeriana officinalis

Parts used: Root.

Properties/Actions: Sedative, relaxing nervine, anticonvulsant, antispasmodic, hypotensive, hypnotic, anodyne, carminative.

Benefits: Eases restlessness, insomnia, hysteria, anxiety, hyperactivity, cramps, backaches, emotional stress.

Used effectively for sleeplessness associated with pain.

Suggested uses: Tincture, capsules.

Growing, harvesting, and wild crafting tips and specifics: Perennial. Plant from root divisions, or start from seed indoors or in the greenhouse, late winter or early spring, transplant into the garden after danger of frost. When taking or giving root divisions for yours or a friend's garden, take from the outer edges—the roots form a crown underground and are least disturbed with this kind of division.

Full sun to partial shade is ideal, and any type of relatively well-drained soil will do.

Cautions: May increase sleeping time, or leave a groggy feeling in the morning if the dose is too high, or if taken late in the night versus before going to bed.

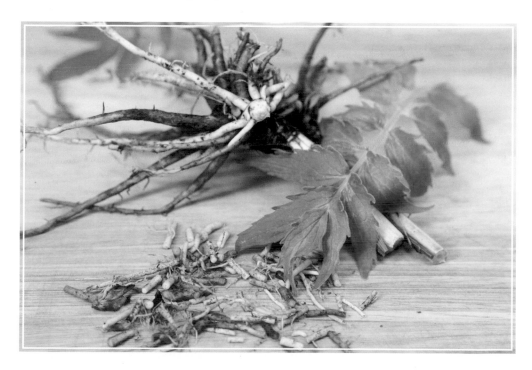

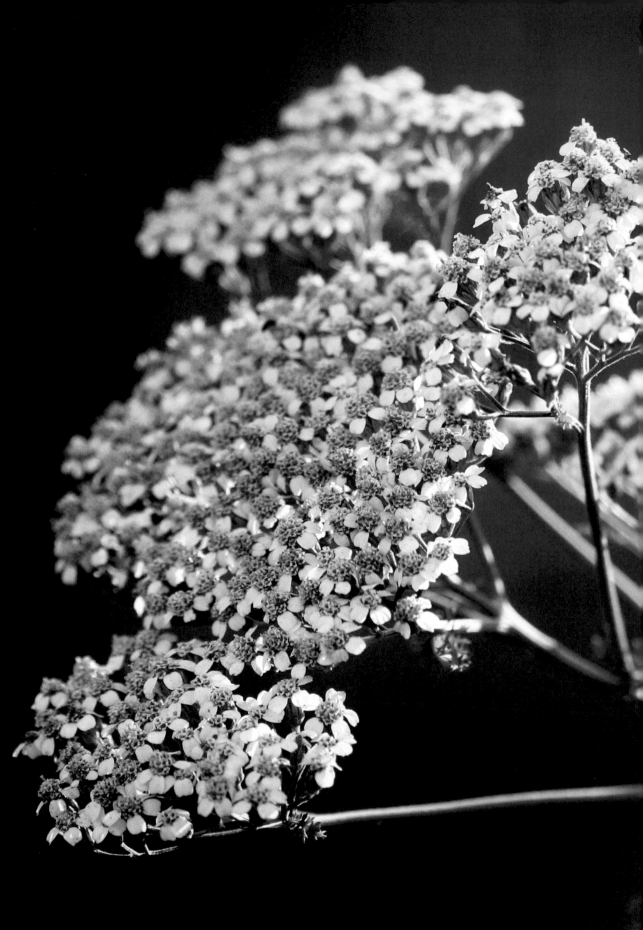

Yarrow
Achillea millefolium

Parts used: Flowers, leaves, stems.

Properties/Actions: Diaphoretic, anti-inflammatory, anti-pyretic, antispasmodic, stomachic, astringent, carminative, hemostatic.

Benefits: Beneficial for colds, flus, fevers, bleeding, hemorrhoids, suppressed menses, and hypertension.

Yarrow is very well-known for use in "sweating out" a fever. Great in an infusion combined with elder blossoms, lemon balm, and peppermint at the onset of a cold or flu, to keep it moving through you, in order to speed healing.

Very effective in stopping bleeding when the powder is directly applied. Long associated as first aid for the battlefield, and thus named after the warrior Achilles.

Suggested uses: Infusion, tincture, powder.

Growing, harvesting, and wild crafting tips and specifics: Grows wild in fields and forest edges all summer long. Harvest when flowers are in their prime—the beginning of the blooming period. Likes full sun, and drier conditions.

Cautions: Can cause profuse sweating, and can raise a fever too much if consumed in high quantities.

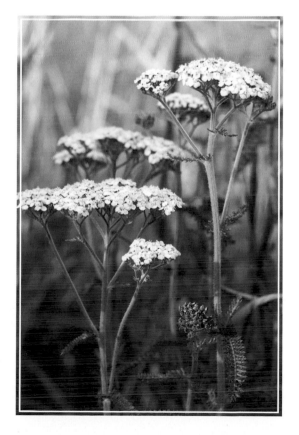

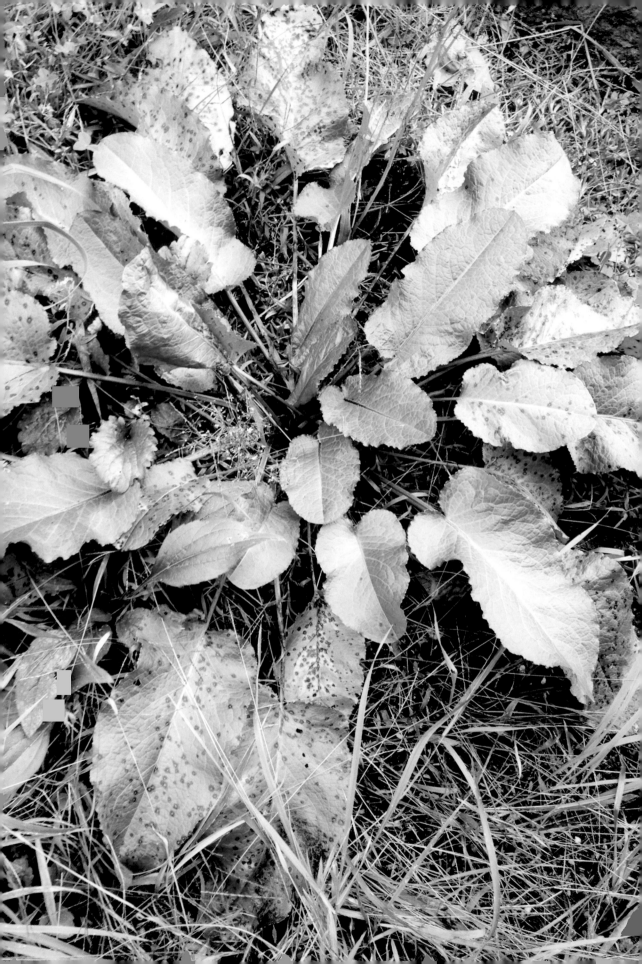

Yellow Dock
Rumex crispus

Parts used: Root.

Properties/Actions: Nutritive, alterative, mild laxative, blood tonic, cholagogue.

Benefits: Beneficial for anemia, skin diseases including eczema, psoriasis, acne, herpes, liver congestion, gall bladder disorders, and gastrointestinal diseases.

Suggested Uses: Tincture, decoction, syrup

Growing, harvesting, and wild crafting tips and specifics: Perennial. Grows along roadsides, in wetter areas, often growing alongside burdock and dandelion. Does well in sun or shade.

Cautions: None at this time.

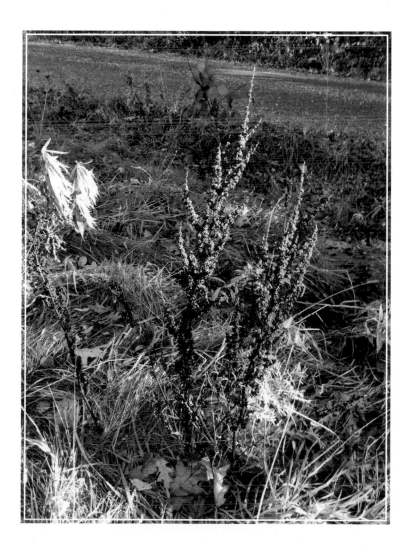

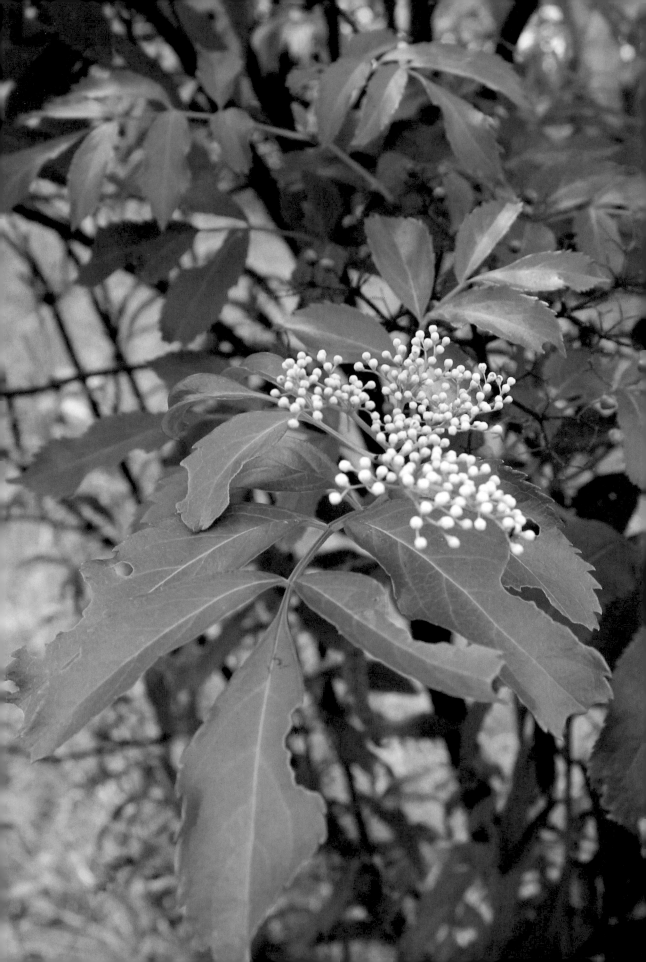

CULTIVATING THE MEDICINAL GARDEN

There are so many reasons to plant an herb garden or incorporate herbs into a vegetable garden. In addition to the health benefits, herbs serve as great companions for vegetables—their strong scent wards off pests—and they are beautiful growing in the garden or cut for flower arrangements.

This book's methods and cultivation techniques are most applicable to a temperate climate, which is defined as having four distinguishable seasons with winters cold enough to force the ground to freeze (below 32 degrees Fahrenheit and 10 degrees Celsius). The map provided below shows the various zones in North America.

There are so many ways to customize the growing of herbs for your specific situation—whether it be a small garden right outside the kitchen door with mostly edibles, a large herb/veggie garden in your backyard, or potted herbs on your deck or in/on the windowsill.

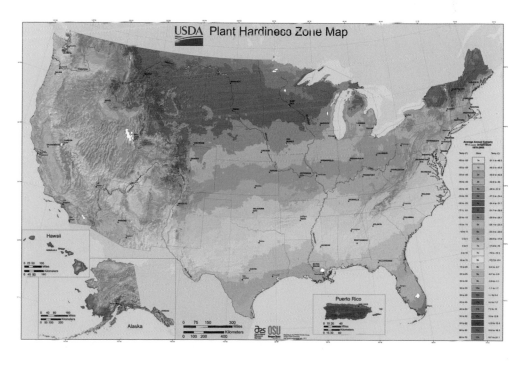

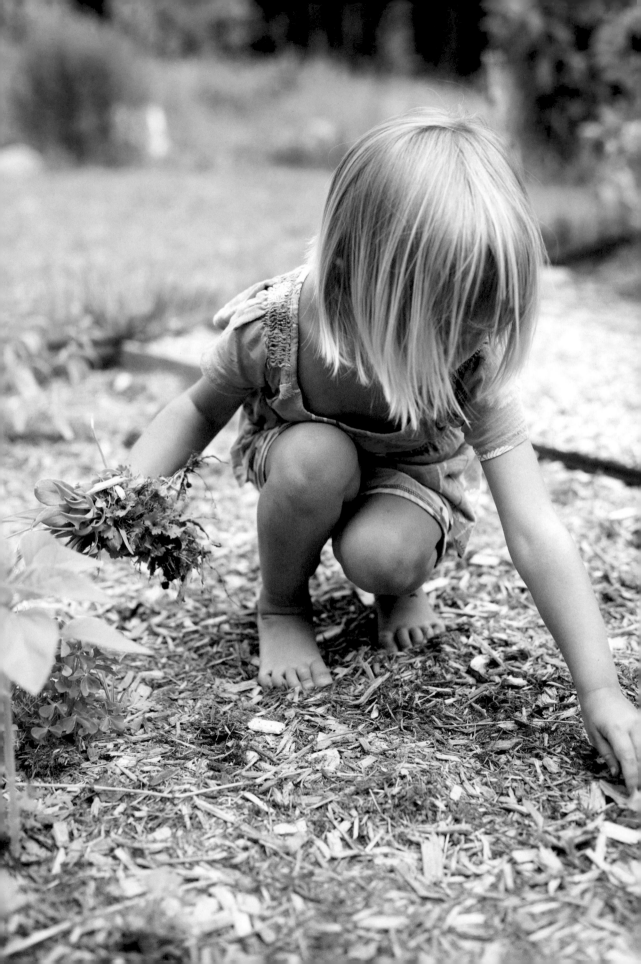

In this section, we will discuss designs, locations, soil types, drainage, fertilizer, mulch, weeds, planting roots, seeds, cuttings, preparing the ground for planting, tools, time of year for planting, and choosing herbs to plant that suit your needs. For the urban gardener, or for those of you who do not have a piece of ground to devote to herbs, we will provide information on how to grow herbs in pots or planters, either inside or out.

There are many ways to arrange your gardens depending on what your goals are. Start by thinking about what plants you'd like to grow and utilize for what purposes.

Choosing the herbs to grow

The first step is to choose the herbs to plant that will be your healing allies for either a season, or for years to come.

Think about what ails you, in what ways you need or want to feel better, what illnesses are prevalent in your family, and what herbs you would like to have on hand for cooking, for first aid, for aromatherapy. Which herbs from the list and beyond call to you, intrigue you, or seem like fun to grow.

Brainstorm, dream, sketch, and think about the medicines or body care products you'd like to be able to reach for in your cabinet in times of need.

When thinking about planting the garden, the first step is to consider annuals, biennials, and perennials. Perennials are herbs that will keep coming back year after year if properly protected through the winter and are hardy to the place you live. These plants will spread. Biennials will produce every two years. Annuals will grow for one year only, so there is more room for experimentation here. Lets take a look at some of the plants on our list:

Astragalus	Perennial
Boneset	Perennial
Burdock	Biennial
Calendula	Annual
Chamomile	Annual
Comfrey	Perennial
Dandelion	Biennial
Echinacea	Perennial
Elder	Perennial
Garlic	Annual
Lavender	Perennial
Lemon balm	Perennial
Motherwort	Perennial
Mugwort	Perennial
Mullein	Biennial
Peppermint	Perennial
Plantain	Perennial
Red clover	Perennial
Red raspberry	Perennial
Sage	Perennial
Self-heal	Perennial
St. John's wort	Perennial
Valerian	Perennial
Yellow dock	Perennial

As you can see, most of these are perennials. Here are a few more examples of herbs that are annuals that you can try out year to year until you find the ones you love to grow and use: rosemary, oats, parsley, basil and tulsi (holy) basil. All annuals may self-seed themselves, naturally giving you more of them the following year and therefore acting like perennials, but this cannot be counted on.

There are also all the wild wonderful medicinal weeds that grow all around us in our lawns and forest edges and fields. Keep in mind that there is always the option of incorporating them into your garden. If there are wild plants that you love and are not easily found around where you live, or if you are in a more urban area, it may be a good idea!

A short list of some options here: St. John's wort, yellow dock, red raspberry, mullein, mushrooms, red clover, dande-lion, yarrow, nettle.

Herb garden designs

Once you have a good idea what plants you will be growing and have chosen a site for your garden, designing the garden is in order. Before turning ground, making beds, and adding compost and other amendments, designing on paper is a good idea. Think about what shape you want, what size, whether to do raised beds or not, etc. Here are some drawings of design options to get the creative thinking going.

Herb gardens can be very simply designed or very intricate. Think of your garden as an empty palette where you can mix and match colors and moods and reflections to your own individual needs and desires. Another way to consider the layout of your garden is to imagine your-self sculpting the earth. You are an earth sculptor!

Here are a couple of unique possibili-ties to get the creative juices flowing.

Moon Garden

A moon garden is a garden bed shaped like a crescent moon, with a couple of walkways for access. The moon garden could include plants that are used for women's moon cycles and/or plants that display whitish leaves and white flowers. Enjoying a moon garden is easy: one can walk through the garden at night and take in the view, especially if the moon is out. According the *Farmer's Almanac* the age-old practice of performing farm chores by the moon stems from the simple belief that the moon governs moisture. Pliny the Elder, the first-century Roman naturalist, stated in his *Natural History* that the moon "replenishes the earth; when she approaches it, she fills all bodies, while, when she recedes, she empties them."

Mandala Garden

A mandala garden is a series of garden beds set up in a circular fashion. In one example, the beds are arranged splaying out from the middle of a circle. Plants of specific colors are in certain places, with specific plants blooming at certain times. Traditionally in the small backyard herb garden, the perennials form the structure or "skeleton" of the garden and the annuals fill in around them. Annuals are planted each year, and so there are times where areas are bare, either before planting or after harvesting. This general design keeps the garden feeling full, even when there are no annuals growing. Perennials grow bigger each year, so leaving plenty of room around them for spreading is important.

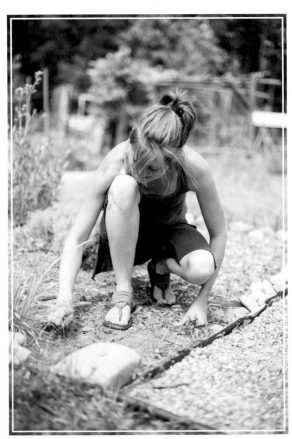

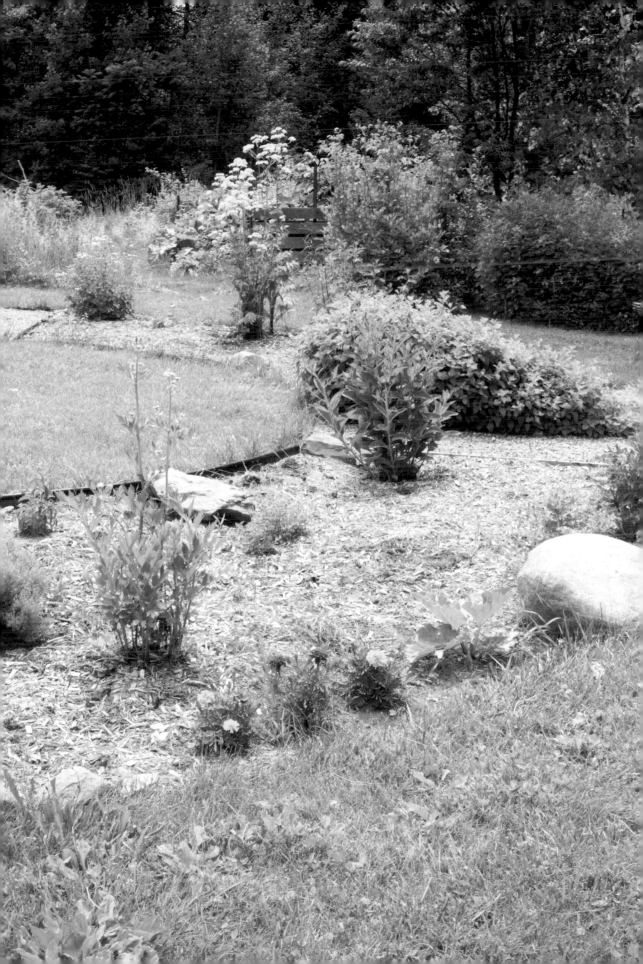

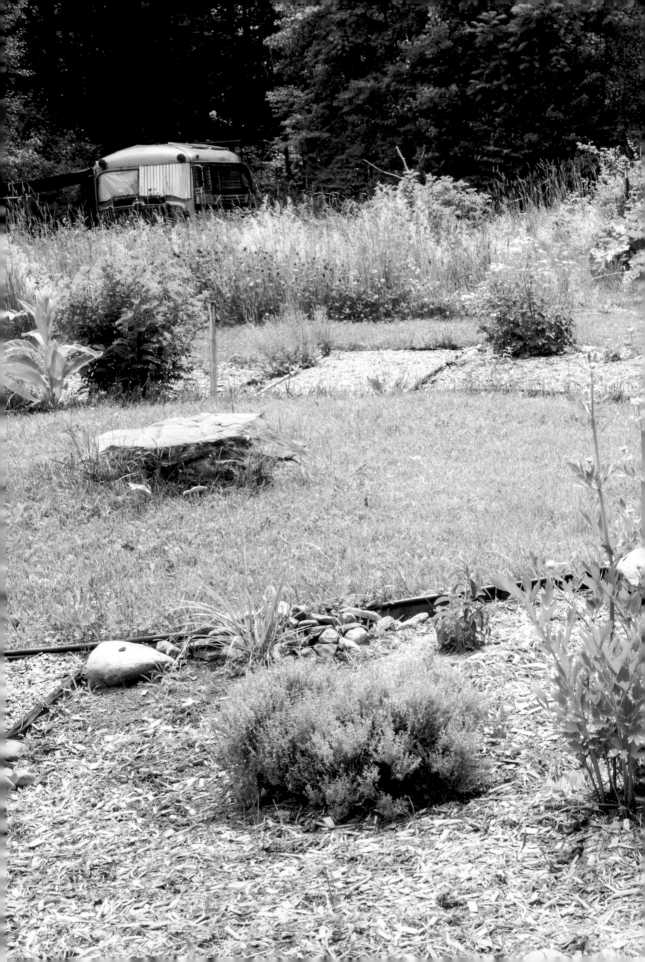

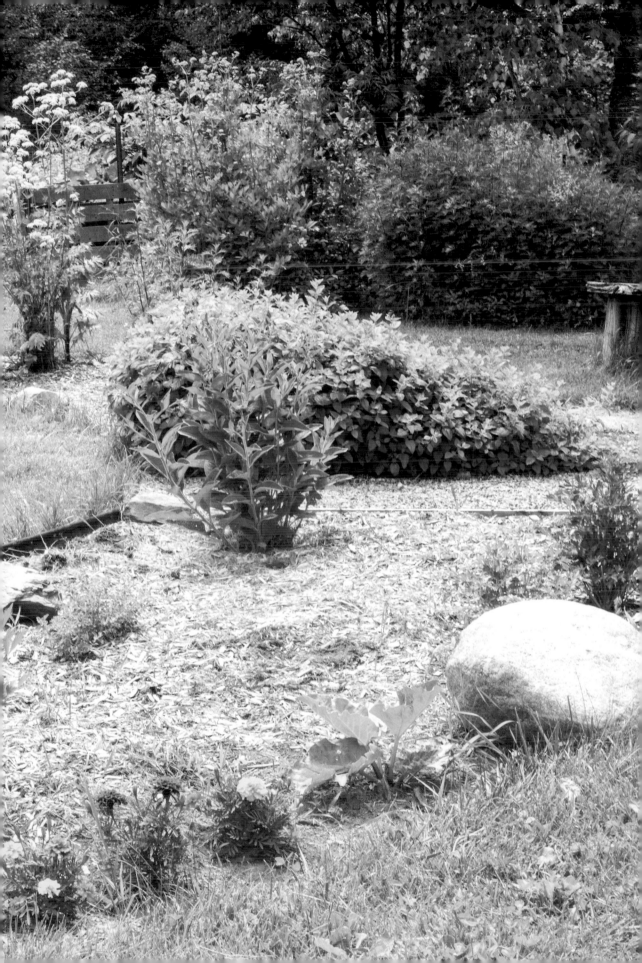

Medicine Wheel Garden

A medicine wheel garden is a circular garden, usually divided into four quadrants, one for each of the four compass directions. The four directions have many representations and symbols that correspond with them in many cultures around the world.

As a simple example, East represents new life, birth, beginnings, and morning. South represents fire, heat, the middle of life, and passion. North represents the elder years, coldness, and winter. West represents the end of the day, sleep, rejuvenation, and death.

These are just some representations that I have taken from various traditions (mostly earth-based spirituality) and incorporated into my intention when designing and planting my medicine wheel garden.

After you have done your own research on medicine wheels around the world, looked into the symbolism of the four directions, and thought about what is meaningful to you—maybe from your heritage or rituals and symbols that resonate with you—then you can start connecting the plants to them. Consider all of these things, as well as the size of your gardening space, and then choose your plants. This type of garden is meant to be a sacred space, an art project really. It is enjoyable to create something that is so customized to you and to really make it your own.

Herbs (especially perennials) spread, so make sure to leave plenty of space around each one, and cover the ground between them with either wood chip mulch or straw or whatever else you like. Here are some ideas for coordinating plants and compass directions:

For the East: motherwort, calendula, sage, lavender, catnip, St. John's wort.

For the South: echinacea, thyme, boneset, astragalus.

For the North: parsley, lemongrass, oregano, basil, rhubarb.

For the West: valerian, lemon balm, chamomile, feverfew, holy basil.

These herbs, for me personally, correspond with the directions as I mentioned earlier. They are used in different stages of life, as well as different times of day.

Along with planting herbs in the medicine wheel garden, it's fun to also collect many stones to place around, perhaps making a border with them, as well as stumps to sit on, a grassy area in the middle, an altar of some sort in the middle, prayer flags, etc. The options are endless—have fun with it!

If you want to dive deep into the world of medicine wheels and learn how to incorporate them into your life, I recommend *The Medicine Wheel Garden: Creating Sacred Space for Healing, Celebration, and Tranquility* by E. Barrie Kavasch.

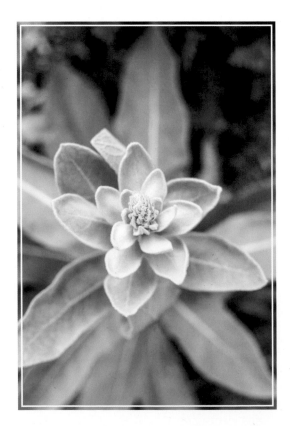

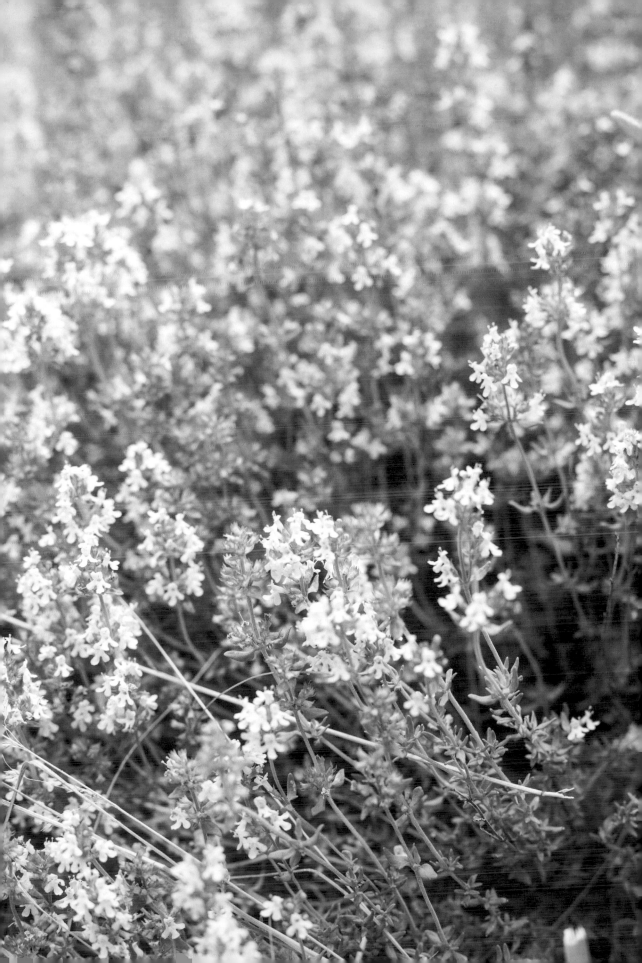

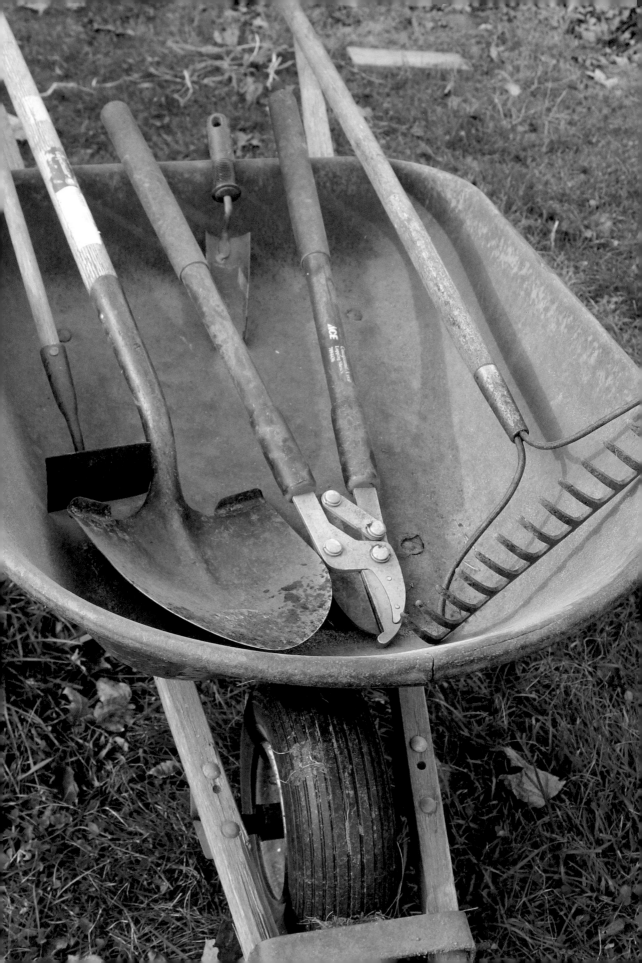

Implementing the Medicinal Herb Garden

Tools you will need

Whether you are digging into sodded ground or planting in prepared soil, there are some basic tools you will need to have on hand.

- **Garden spade shovel**—Choose a spade that is sharp and sturdy enough to dig through sod and turn soil for planting. If you were using a tractor, you would plow the ground first, before tilling it for planting. The shovel is used to "plow" by hand. You and your shovel turn over large clumps of ground, and it can be quite a workout!
- **Garden or "rock" rake**—This is a heavy duty steel, short-tined rake for raking rocks, clumps of weeds, grass, sod, or brambles out of your area. Also used for smoothing out the garden beds to ready them for planting, after they are prepared.
- **Hoe**—A hoe is used for hilling up soil and weeding. It comes in handy especially in the beginning for building garden beds. Once an area is dug up, all the sod taken away if need be, and close to rock free, you can go around and create beds with the hoe by hilling soil away from where you want pathways, and onto the areas that will be for planting. There are a few different styles of hoes: the stirrup hoe, which is essentially a metal "stirrup" on the end of the wooden handle, is great for getting underneath the roots of weeds and pulling them up, without moving too much soil around. This type is better for weeding than hilling generally. Then there are different sizes of the traditional type hoe. A large traditional hoe works best for helping to make garden beds. There are also crook-neck hoes, an older type that serves the same purpose. Finally, there are hand hoes, which are great for weeding and furrowing. It's nice to have a couple different sizes and types around.
- **Gloves**—Gloves are especially important if you are preparing an area where there are brambles or poison ivy, or the like. There are endless varieties and sizes of garden gloves, leather being the most durable, but not always the most comfortable. Another reason to wear gloves is to protect your hands from getting dry and/or cracked from working with the soil.
- **Spade**—A small garden spade is helpful for digging holes to plant seedlings, or to dig/cut perennials out of the ground by separating them to plant in another place or give away.
- **Clippers, large and small**—Clippers are used to cut plants back (prune), and/or harvest. When clearing an area, there may be plants—namely brambles—that you need to cut back before digging the roots from the ground. There are long-handled clippers for getting the larger and harder to reach plants, and short-handled ones for smaller, more accessible plants.
- **Rototiller™**—A Rototiller is a machine that you walk behind and push that tills the ground for you! It's used to make non-raised beds. If used many times in the same spot, a rototiller may create a bed pan: a hardening down of the soil right underneath the soil that is tilled, thus making it hard for roots to grow deep.

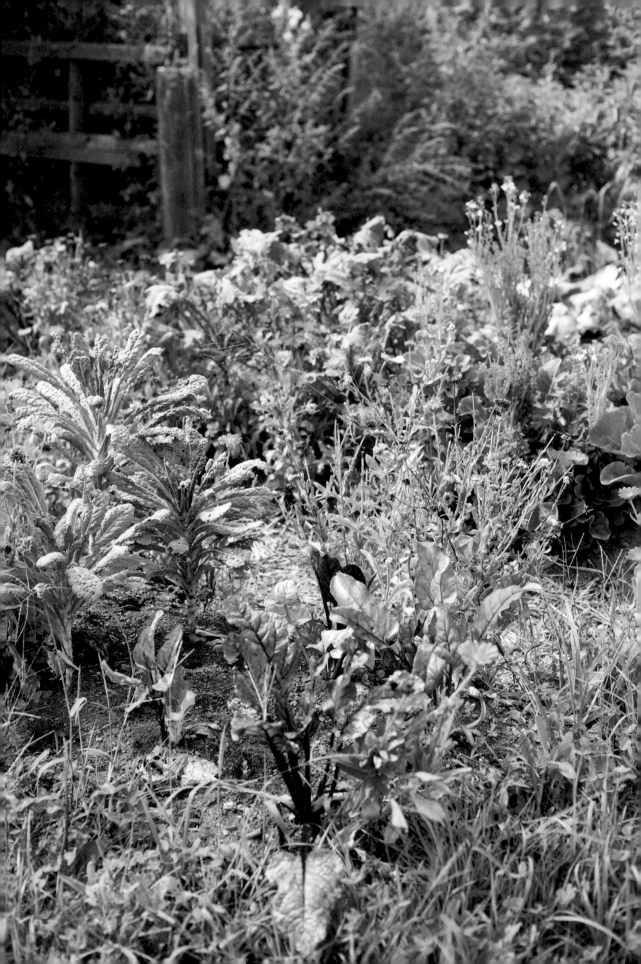

Preparing an area for planting

Raised Beds

Raised beds are garden beds that are raised above the surrounding ground. There are a few reasons they are nice: they are easier to access for weeding, pruning, and harvesting and they allow better drainage to prevent the area from becoming waterlogged. They can also be very attractive, especially if you build them up with stones or wood.

Raised beds can be very simple and newly dug each year. These are the kind that are built up with materials such as stones or wood, which create a more permanent structure of a bed. Not only do they look good, they also function to hold in the soil, thus preventing erosion.

With a bed that does not have a border of stone or wood, it's usually only slightly raised, so you'll need to bend down to the ground to weed, use a hoe, or dig with a shovel. If the bed is really high, and surrounded by stone or wood, you can sit on the edge, or bend over slightly to weed, and do the work that needs to be done—usually with a small garden spade or hand hoe.

When building raised beds of any type, if you have nice topsoil already on your location you can just dig it and use it. Alternatively, you may need to have some delivered. If you're building the bed up high, build the frame, and then shovel or pour the soil right in, along with other desired materials such as leaves to fluff it up and compost to increase fertility.

Raised beds can be very beautiful and defined or just small mounded areas.

Instructions for making raised beds

If you are starting out with a lawn or field, you'll need to remove the sod and/or grass and weeds. Take your long-handled shovel, and start digging! As you are turning clumps and shaking as much soil out as possible, removing the sod and weeds, this material can then be collected and composted. Keep a wheelbarrow nearby to collect the compostable material.

Now that you have cleared and dug a little, and it's starting to look like a potential garden, it's time to "sculpt" the garden. Wherever you want a bed for planting, dig along the edges of that area, and transfer the soil from around the edges into the middle, thus starting to distinguish the beds from the pathways.

A bed filled with plants should be no wider than 5 feet maximum, so that you can reach the middle from both sides for planting, weeding, harvesting, etc.

Once you have made your bed (simple raised bed, not built up with a border), and have ample pathways around it, it is the time to add soil amendments if needed (see later in this section). Whatever recipe you choose, mix it in thoroughly. It's also a good idea to mulch the pathways with straw, leaves, thickly laid hay, or woodchips, to prevent weeds from creeping into the garden beds.

To make raised beds with stones around them, collect stones of whatever size and shape you have or can find close by. Perhaps there are stones you can collect from a nearby river, or by the ocean to remind you of trips you have taken.

If you have no stones, buying them from a stone retailer or stone worker is an option. Build a stone wall that will

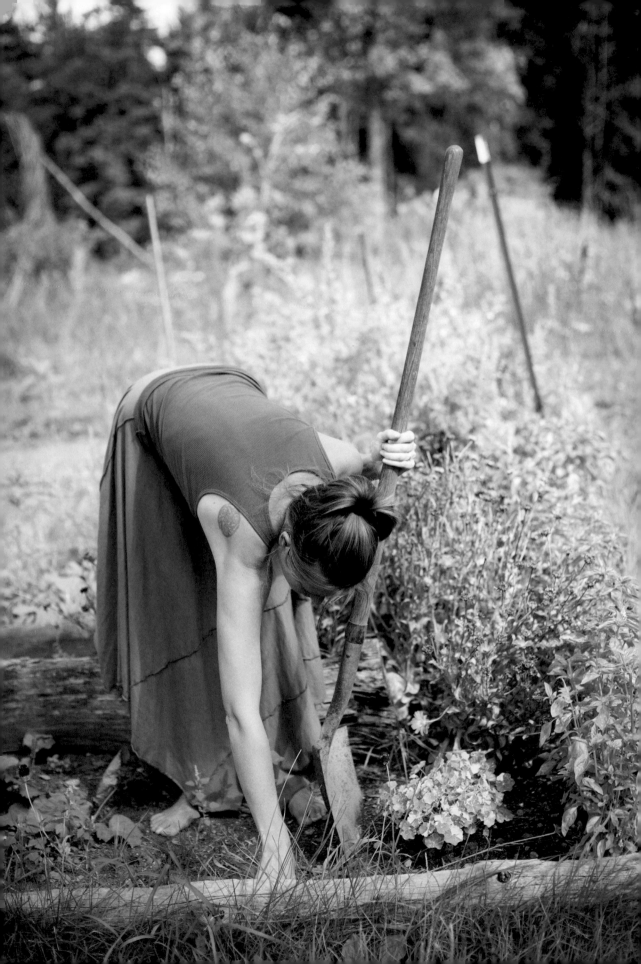

enclose the bed, as high as desired, and fill with soil and amendments. You can also build the bed up first and then build the wall around it, but most likely you will still need to fill it in at the end to top it off.

If you are set on plans for building a wooden raised bed, you can follow the simple instructions here.

Non-raised beds

Non-raised beds are defined as areas that are dug down with pathways around them. Just dig down into the ground and add soil amendments! These beds tend to be a little more easily compacted, and it's important to be sure that there is plenty of top soil so that you are not planting into subsoil—which is very dense and since it is void of nutrients, not much likes to grow in it. You can always build up these beds just by adding materials such as leaves or straw and compost, which will get incorporated into the soil on the flat ground and will eventually decompose and create more fluffy soil in the beds each year.

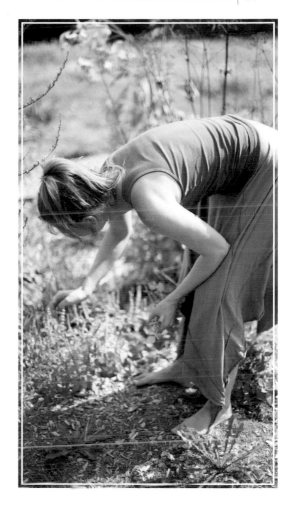

Get boards (never pressure-treated because the chemicals used to preserve the wood will leech into your soil and therefore into your plants via the roots), ideally cedar or locust because they will last a long time without rotting. Make a box where your bed will be! No bottom or top— just the sides—and nail or screw the boards together and fill in with soil and amendments.

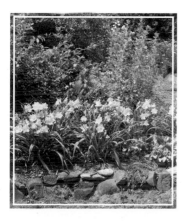
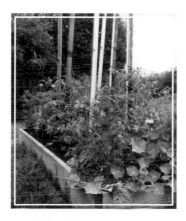
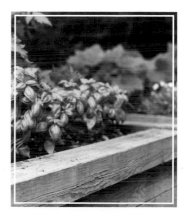

Deep-dug bed method (or "double digging")

The deep-dug bed method is to dig a very deep garden bed just once and never walk on it or put any weight on it again. Deep-dug beds allow you to grow up to four times more plants in a space, which makes it extremely useful if you are working with a small space to grow in.

The other reason for this method is that the roots of the plants will grow down deeper, and while taking up less space sideways, the plants will be bigger and maybe happier—and depending on which plants you use, they will have more room to spread out.

This method is more often used for growing vegetables than just herbs, but we have included instructions here because many of you will be growing both vegetables and herbs alongside each other.

Instructions to Dig the Deep Bed

Dig a spade's depth (garden shovel with long handle) and put soil aside on the ground right next to the bed. Now dig down another spade's depth to loosen the soil beneath. Add a large amount of manure—two scoops per square foot—then put the soil you set aside back on top. Keep going like this until you have the bed the size and shape you want. Plant into it, and never tread on it. This is a one-time job; you will never have to dig the bed again, so essentially, it then becomes a no-till bed over time. With this method, you can plant your vegetables or herbs closer together. There is no space too small to grow herbs and vegetables in!

No-till method

No-till means no turning of the soil. In different regions and climates, this can be done in different ways. Some plants do well with this method, some not so much.

In temperate climates, things break down more slowly, because winter interrupts the process of decay each year. Using a sheet mulching technique works well to mimic nature, creating a humus layer on the top of the ground that is welcoming to new plant starts, and seeds. The key is to create fluffy beds, without digging down and turning.

Sheet mulching starts by laying something on your garden bed that will kill the grass and weeds that are there. Newspapers, cardboard, or even old rugs or blankets (make sure they are nontoxic) will work well. Collecting cardboard and/or newspapers takes time, but usually you can get quite a few for free from grocery stores, gas stations, etc.—places that are needing to get rid of them and are happy for you to take them away. To prepare them for the garden, make sure to take off all tape and labels and the glossy parts from the newspapers. Break down the boxes to make them flat.

Next, cover the area by overlapping materials so that no grass is peeking through. Now comes a layer of mulch. Leaves in the fall are a really good mulching option. They decompose rapidly, making for light, fluffy soil within one season. Straw or hay takes a little longer to decompose and is usually more expensive. If you don't have your own leaves in your yard to rake up and apply, collect them from around town! People leave them in leaf bags for pick up at the end of their driveways, and these are free for the taking.

- Mulch hay sometimes is free, especially if partially rotted, and farmers may be looking to give it away.
- Straw is nice to add fluff, and can be purchased at farm stores or nurseries.
- Grass clippings are okay, but will get slimy quickly if left not mixed in thoroughly with other drier materials, so make sure to do this.
- Manure, composted manure, and your own food scrap compost are ingredients to be incorporated into your sheet mulching operation. Again, these are materials you either have on hand or need to obtain. Try for organic.

Once you have all your materials, start layering them over your base layer of cardboard or the like. Ideally make each layer as thick as possible, and alternate between dry and wet materials. An example: cardboard, manure, leaves, grass clippings, leaves, manure, straw.

To test if your layers of mulch have broken down, reach down through with your hand and feel what's down there. If it's soil-like, and if there are worms in it, you can plant!

If you are using this technique and planting perennials (echinacea, astragalus, etc.), you will only go through this process once, to set up the garden initially. Each year after, you will just mulch with various materials—all the ones we've mentioned except cardboard—in order to keep the plants fertilized and healthy and to keep weeds down around them.

For annuals (such as chamomile, garlic, calendula, etc.), the beds will be cleared out by pulling up the plants and composting them or chopping them up and leaving them in the bed, and new mulch added to rebuild the beds each year. You will come up with your own mulching recipes!

Most likely you will have beds comprised of a combination of annuals and perennial, in which case the bulk of the work is done in the first year, and you continue to maintain each year, planting annuals between the perennials, and mulching all around.

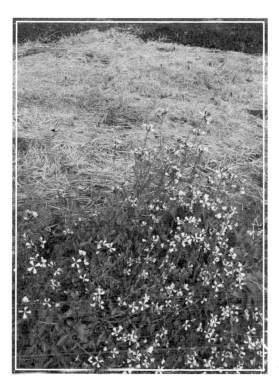

Testing, Soil Types, and Amending Your Soil

There are a number of soil testing "kits" on the market that will show you whether your soil is deficient in nitrogen, phosphorous, potassium, or trace elements. You can also contact your state extension service for testing. Though herbs will thrive in nearly any soil, it can be valuable to learn what your soil either is lacking or has too much of, especially if you are planting vegetables along with your herbs. You will learn

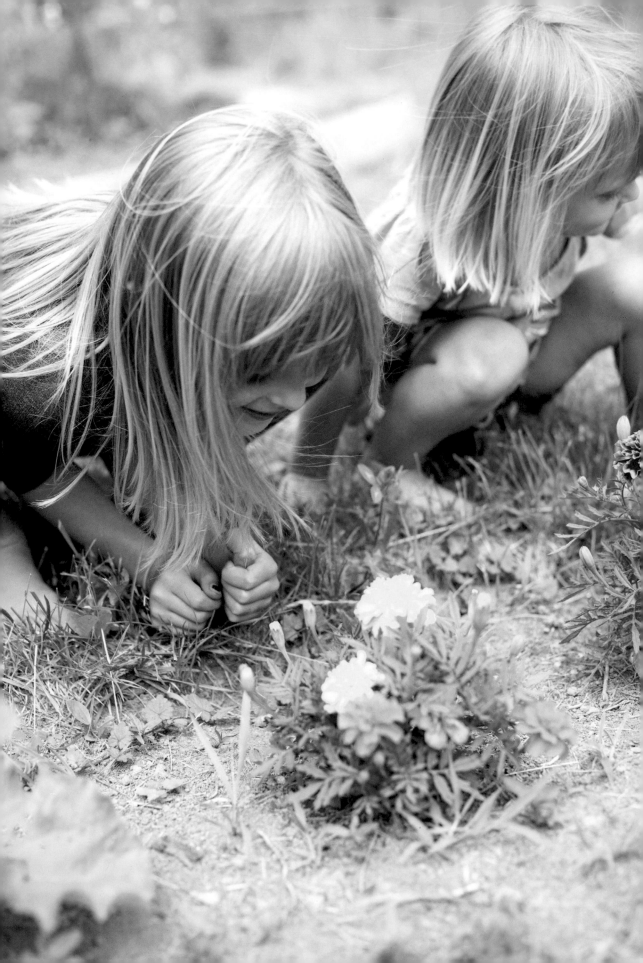

what minerals and other nutrients exist in what quantities, and from there be able to decipher what (if any) amendments can be added to help plants grow better.

Often even more important than knowing the exact nutrients in the soil is the consistency—whether it's sandy, loamy, or clay-like. The goal is to get a nice fluffy loam—somewhere between sand and clay—that is filled with life and nutrients. The main way to improve the consistency of any soil and to create a living environment is to be always adding humus. Humus is everything that soil should be, and it is made by adding anything to the soil that was or is alive. These materials are the ones we've talked about in the no-till method section as well as the list of amendments below, and are always things we mulch with regardless of whether we have tilled the garden or not. Anything we put on the top of the soil will be incorporated by the worms and other living things. Humus is really the basis of good soil, and therefore a good garden. Without it, things would not grow without the use of chemicals.

Each plant has a unique set of conditions in which it will thrive best. Our job, when planting a garden, is to find a way to make the most plants the happiest by creating soil that is a neutral pH, not too acidic, and not too alkaline. Luckily, herbs are pretty flexible with soil type (see the Meet the Plants section for details on ideal growing conditions for each plant).

Some soil amendments and what they do are:

- Bone meal: concentrated minerals
- Blood meal: very concentrated form of nitrogen
- Fish emulsion: adds nitrogen and minerals
- Compost or manure: adds nitrogen, prevents excess alkalinity

- Lime (crushed limestone): remedies excess acidity
- Peat (peat moss): aerates the soil
- Seaweed: adds minerals and nitrogen

Planting Your Garden

This section includes general modes of planting herbs. For details on specific plants see the Meet the Plants section.

From seed

Direct seeding herbs right into the soil works better for some plants than others. Starts (seeds that have sprouted and are beginning to grow) are more likely to take to the garden bed and thrive than straight seeds, which are vulnerable to an herb or insect gobbling them up, or the conditions not being ideal because of the unpredictability of the weather or animals running over the beds and messing them up. There are some instances though when direct seeding is the best, or can at least work moderately well—especially for fast-growing annuals like calendula or basil.

Sometimes mindfully placing the seeds about 6 inches apart is called for, and other times just scattering them about is fine—especially if you want a thick bed of something, like mint or lemon balm.

Seeds can be started inside your home in flats or pots or in a greenhouse. Many herb seeds need to be established far before the growing season outside is appropriate and the danger of frost is over. Each particular herb will have directions on the packet as to how it needs to be started, and often other tips on ideal growing conditions.

Some seeds need special treatment, like scarification, or being frozen for a length of time. And some herbs are nearly impossible to start from seed, so cuttings or divided roots are better methods.

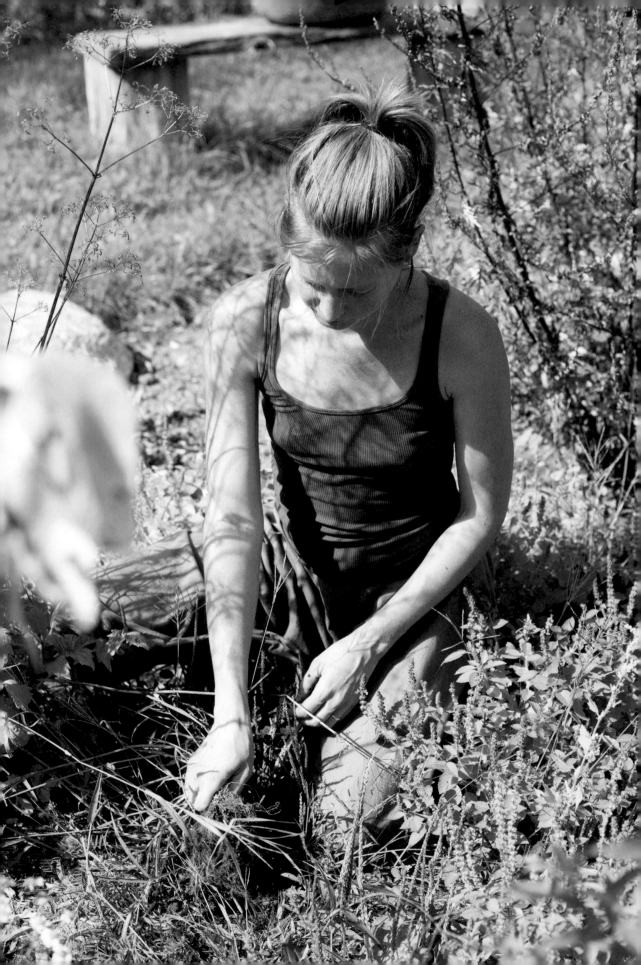

From starts (young plants)

Starts are plants that are already established in small pots of soil and are ready for planting directly into your garden when the conditions are right.

You can either get the starts going from seed at home in a window or greenhouse, or get them at the farmer's market or from a nursery. Make sure to space the plants properly, at least six inches apart, often more, to ensure plenty of room for growth over the season—and for perennials, over many seasons to come.

Many of the more common herbs are easy to find as starts, but some are harder to source depending on where you live (see sources).

From cuttings

Some herbs you can take cuttings from, others you can't. The way to take a cutting is to cut off a nice healthy piece of the plant you would like to propagate.

The key is to sprout the end you've cut in water. If it sprouts well, you can then plant it, and hope that the roots take off. (See the prior section on Meet the Plants for specific plants that grow well from cuttings.)

From divided roots

In the fall or the spring, when you are harvesting roots, you can take some and move them around, to spread them and make new garden patches! This can be fun—you can have perennial swaps with friends. This only works with perennial herbs, and you only want to take roots and divide them for planting after the plant has been established for at least three years.

Dig down and get some roots, while trying not to disturb the rest of the plant. Break it apart, shake off the soil (or not), and keep moist until you are ready to plant it again.

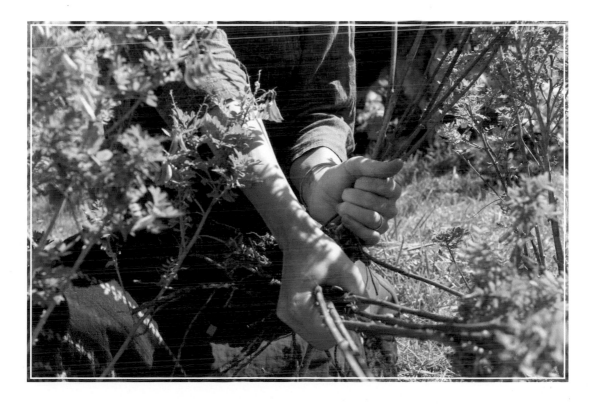

Planting from divided roots is the most common and easy way to deal with perennial herbs. Seek out people in and around your community who have gardens, and it might turn out to be easy to get all the plants you want to grow for free! Especially with herbs like comfrey or mint that spread like crazy, people are often looking to pass some along.

Weeding

What a rewarding task it is to free our herbal friends from the confines of unwanted imposters. A "weed" is simply a misplaced plant. Often the weeds are medicinal plants, and so when going along clearing them away from the ones you planted, you may keep them for medicine, or just return them to the earth or compost pile.

If we are cultivating something it is important that we give it space to grow. The easiest time to pull the weeds is when they are young and delicate and have not yet established strong roots or gone to seed. The roots of some weeds are hard to obtain, and so digging down all the way to get all of them out can be difficult, and sometimes not worth it. We can always go back and try again. Having areas more densely planted with plants we want and also mulching are two ways to prevent rampant weeds. The more bare soil we provide, the more the weeds will come in and make it their home. Who can blame them?

Insect control

Herb gardens don't have many pests! And vegetable gardens that have a lot of herbs incorporated into them don't have as many pests as straight vegetable gardens.

Herbs themselves are insect repellents, so this section is pretty short! The main thing to keep in mind to prevent unwanted plant-eating bugs in any garden is the health of the garden and each individual plant. The healthier the garden, the less likely insects will attack. So feeding your garden soil the nutrients it needs to thrive and produce (mostly with compost), and keeping it weed free and watered when necessary, are the main things to do to manage pests. Planting different kinds of plants in the same area—mimicking nature in this way—will also help to ward off pests naturally.

If there are only a few pests in your garden, you don't need to do anything aggressive. Using a chemical pest deterrent disrupts the delicate balance of life, often creating a dependency on the chemical. Even homemade sprays like cayenne pepper or diluted soapy water can be potentially damaging, and usually unnecessary.

Garlic, yarrow, calendula, and all varieties of marigold, valerian, thyme, wormwood, rosemary, and sage are all standbys. They are great to have here and there throughout any garden to keep it protected from many pests, and to help vegetables grow bigger and stronger in many cases!

Watering

Watering depends on weather. Sometimes your garden can go a whole year without you needing to give it water. Herbs are resilient, and can live through a lot of adversity.

In general, water the garden if you've had a long dry stretch—a few weeks. If your garden is on the top of a hill, or on a slope, it will dry out faster, and if it's down in a valley, or on the flat ground, it will hold water in the soil longer.

You can water from a hose, a watering can, or a bucket. Be a little more delicate with the more delicate plants and young stages of growth. A stronger stream of

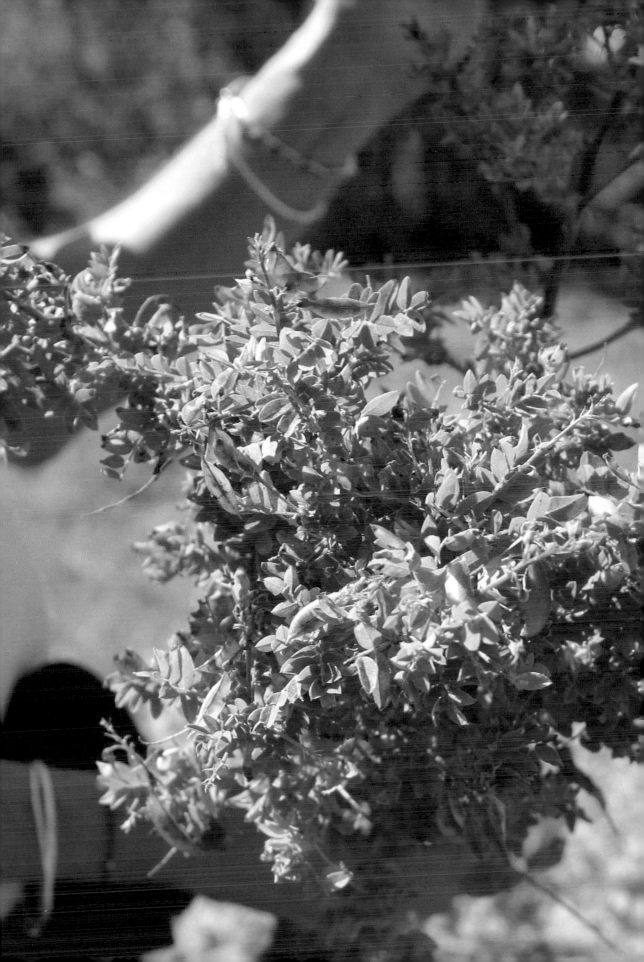

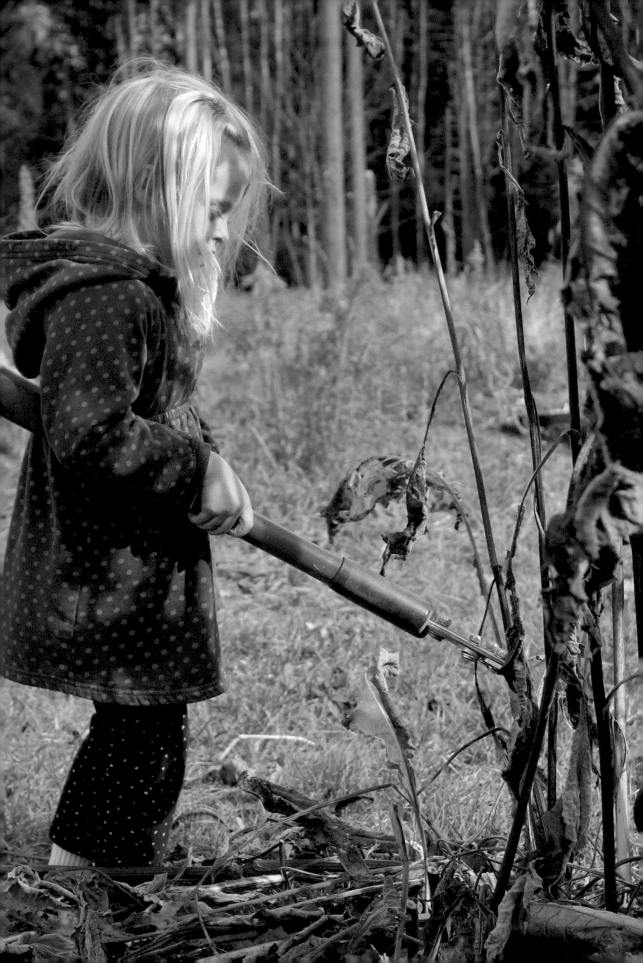

water that is harsh may damage a young plant, so just be aware.

Ideally the water you use on your garden is nice, clean water from a spring or deep well. But, if you only have town or city water, that's what you'll use.

Remember, most herbs are hard to kill, but all herbs will love any extra attention you give them, and will thrive accordingly.

Mulching

Think of the forest for a moment . . . the rich, moist, soft layer of leaves and decaying material makes up the amazing soil that so many plants are thriving in. This environment is nature's mulch system, and is the example we should follow for our gardens. Mulch in the garden keeps weeds from growing, keeps the soil from eroding, brings warmth to the roots for perennials, and ensures rich soil that is being built up by whatever you choose to put on the ground as mulch. Bare soil gets stripped of minerals when it rains; mulched soil is protected.

Materials that can be used as mulch vary depending on the resources that are available to you in your location. Often you can find what you need right on your land, but sometimes you may have to pick up mulch from a neighbor or a store or have loads dropped at your home.

Good mulching materials include leaves, straw, hay, wood chips, compost, spent grain from breweries, pine needles, manure, cardboard, and non-glossy newspapers or paper bags.

Each material will break down at a different speed and provide different nutrients to your soil.

Putting the garden to bed for winter

Ahhh, the end of the growing season is here! After harvesting flowers and leaves of your herbs throughout the spring and summer, and having dug some roots in the fall, it is time to tuck your perennial herbs in for a long winter slumber.

Around late October or early November, it is time to cut back the leftover stems and stalks of perennials. Doing this promotes the downward flow of energy into the roots of the plants and into the ground for hibernation throughout the cold winter months.

Using clippers, clip down the dying plants, chop them up, and put them into the compost. It's nice at this time to take out any last weeds from around the base of the plants. Put some composted manure on, as well as some mulch such as leaves or straw or hay, building up the garden bed 6–12 inches. This will ensure your plants are snug and will be warm for the cold months to come.

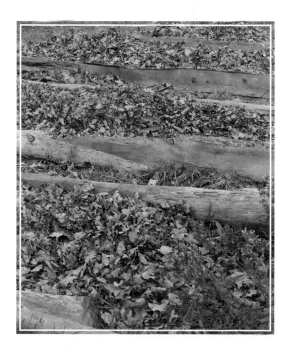

In the spring you will pull some of the mulch away and discover that the compost has mixed with the old soil from the spring rains and the frosting and thawing that has gone on, and new growth will be welcome.

Fall time, around the same time that you are putting the plants to bed, is also the time to plant some roots (see the previous section: From Divided Roots) and bulbs, such as garlic (see the profile on garlic in the Meet the Plants section).

The following table shows some examples of companion plants, which are plants that act as natural effective pesticides and/or fertilizers for each other. This list is by no means exclusive, and in each garden there can be different results. Overall, medicinal and culinary herbs are inherently pest-deterrent.

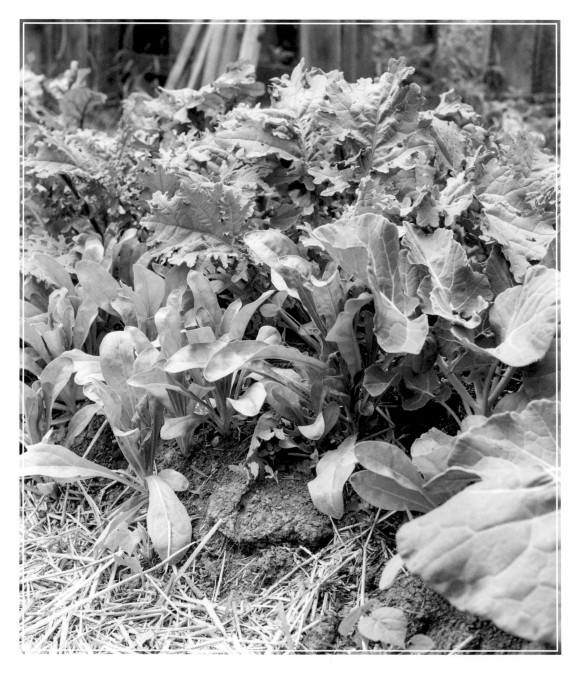

For more in-depth information on companion planting, check out the book *Carrots Love Tomatoes: Secrets of Companion Planting for Successful Gardening* by Louise Riotte.

Vegetable plants and their companion plants

Asparagus:	tomatoes, parsley, basil
Beans:	carrots, cabbage, cucumbers, and many herbs
Beet:	onions
Cabbage family (cabbage, broccoli, kale):	dill, thyme, sage, onions, rosemary, lavender, mint
Carrot:	onions, rosemary, sage, tomatoes, chives, lettuce
Celery:	leeks, cabbage
Corn:	beans, squash
Eggplant:	beans, calendula
Leek:	onions, calendula, carrots, celery
Onion:	lemon balm, marjoram, mint
Potato:	nettle, horseradish, beans, corn, cabbage, mint
Radish:	herbs in general, peas, cucumbers
Spinach:	strawberries
Squash:	calendula, corn, nasturtium
Tomato:	basil, thyme, onion, calendula, chives, carrot
Turnip:	peas

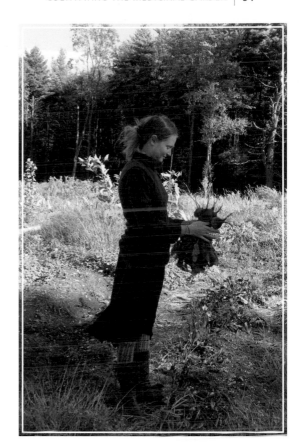

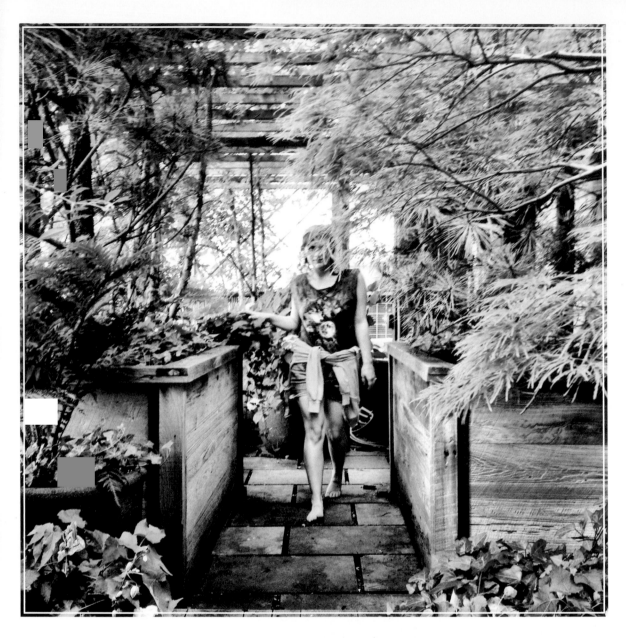
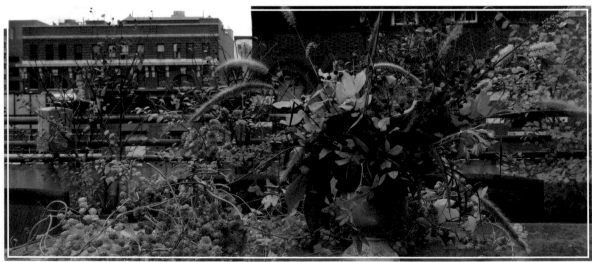

URBAN MEDICINAL GARDENING

The nature of a weed is opportunistic, and we, as humans, have created enormous holes of opportunity for these plants to fill. They have adapted to be at our side, waiting for those favorable times to cover the exposed soils that we continually create. With ever-changing genetics of form, function, and transmutation, weeds have evolved to withstand the punishments that humans unleash upon them.

—Timothy Lee Scott, *Invasive Plant Medicine*

There are so many nooks and crannies in the vast urban areas of the world that can support life—life in the form of medicinal plants! However small your space, if you have the desire to grow some herbs, you can. As we've said earlier, herbs love to grow, and often will do fine with, or even prefer, poor soil and growing conditions. This includes containers on a windowsill, or pots on the deck of your city apartment that gets minimal light and is exposed to poor air quality. Herbs will flourish in containers, and small garden beds between concrete.

Just think about times you have walked the city streets, glancing down at the cracks in the sidewalk, the small piece of earth wedged in along the street and the sidewalk, or the tiny front lawns or abandoned containers with a little soil left in them from the year before. What do you see growing in all of these places? Herbs. They are the plants that take the opportunity to fill the spaces, the cracks.

Some believe that herbs grow where they're needed most, that they seem to "randomly" pop up where their medicine is needed—to either heal the earth, or the people in that area. Take the dandelion for instance; it really is everywhere, and it nourishes our blood, and cleanses our liver, if eaten or taken as a tea or tincture. Wouldn't everyone benefit from acknowledging this amazing medicine, and its incredible diligence to grow, rather than treating it as a weed?

The definition of a weed is a plant that is in the wrong place at the wrong time. While that's true—weeds exist—if

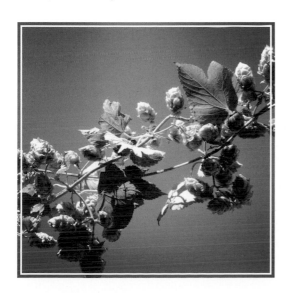

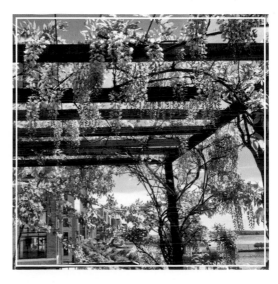

we take a closer look at these weeds, we find that they are useful. It is important to take note that what we think of as common weeds may actually be the medicine we need in our lives. Especially in the city, where not many plants abound, it's important to take note of this dynamic.

When you start opening your eyes to the herbs that are everywhere—even in the most concrete places—it becomes a fun awakening, almost like meeting friends for the first time that were right in front of you your whole life without having noticed them. They are friends from the earth, coming through our barriers, showing us that they will not be stopped; that they have powerful medicine for us, and want to be seen, smelled, and tasted.

Now, when thinking about growing in small spaces in the city, think about that dandelion growing from the tiniest crack in the concrete, and all of a sudden you'll realize how much space you actually have (or can create), to cultivate the herbs you want in and around your home. They will fill your senses with delight, and be very useful in your medicine cabinet all year!

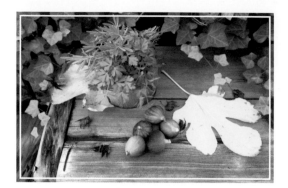

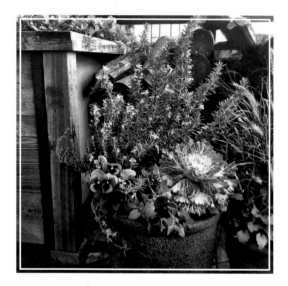

Interview

Courtney Wilder is a Vermonter turned urban landscape gardener. She has been immersed in the world of urban gardening for the past ten years. Courtney grew up with *Healing Herbs* co-author Alyssa Holmes and eagerly spoke to us from her home office in Brooklyn, New York.

AH: Tell us about yourself and how you got into farming, or landscaping, or growing herbs?

CW: Growing up in rural Vermont I was always surrounded by the beauty and the magic of plants. My parents are avid gardeners and I have some other really talented plant ladies that have been in my life since childhood who have inspired me greatly. When I moved to New York City to go to film school, so much of my work was nature inspired. Eventually, when I became disillusioned by the film scene, I started gardening full time. Now I am in this wild niche where I am a private gardener for the very, very wealthy here in Manhattan. I work for myself and I also am part of the garden care team for the landscape design firm Plant Specialists.

AH: Great. Can you tell our readers who are interested in DIY medicinal gardening the different ways and techniques for growing plants in urban areas, or in pots, or on rooftops?

CW: I try to incorporate herbs and edibles into my ornamental planting schemes as much as possible because there are so many that are not only beneficial but also beautiful and aromatic. It's amazing how happy it makes people! They don't even use them necessarily but I think there's something inherent with all of us and [our relationship to] herbs. We feel good when we have herbs near us; it's soothing even for those who are the most out of touch with nature.

Because space is often an issue, even in the most lavish of city homes, I always go small. I use the miniature versions of things like cherry tomatoes, fairy tale eggplants, baby lettuces. With herbs and medicinal plants I'm always looking for things that are interesting as well as useful, like bronze fennel, lemongrass, Queen of Siam basil. I get the smallest-size pots I can, 4 inches ideally, and plant them thickly so that they immediately look beautiful and full without needing tons of soil depth. I avoid herbs that go to seed quickly like cilantro and dill (even though I love them!). When people ask for an herb garden specifically, but don't know what they want, I always start with Simon & Garfunkel's "Scarborough Fair" (parsley, sage, rosemary, and thyme), add basil, and work from there.

AH: That is such a great place for people to start from! There are so many herbs we talk about in this book that can also fit into the beginning-to-plant list (such as calendula, mint, chamomile, and comfrey). Why is it important to grow plants in the city?

CW: Well, personally I would lose my mind without them—plants, whether medicinal or not, teach us about life, death, the seasons. They are always resonating with us on such a low frequency we may not realize it, but they are telling us things. They are telling us about the weather, the environment, the air surrounding us. And they are softening all of our weary eyes in this crazy concrete world.

AH: Since you work primarily with containers and in small spaces, what kind of potting soil do you use?

CW: Sometimes with rooftops there are strict weight restrictions to consider and a really lightweight soil called "Metro Mix" is in order. Usually though, I use a brand called Fafard—it's organic and really good with water retention. Especially when dealing with edibles I only fertilize with a liquid compost or fish emulsion. (Unfortunately, not many people compost in the city.)

AH: Any other tips for our readers who may be just starting out?

CW: It's funny, my first thought was "just plant what you love!" and then I was like wait, that oftentimes is a disaster. You need to know your space. You need to know how much sun you get and how exposed or windy the area is. Then, plant what you love selecting start-up plants that can deal with those conditions. That being said, always experiment, and always buy that weird plant you've never heard of and see what it can do.

AH: Just curious, who are your clients?

CW: Celebrities, heiresses, Wall Street people . . . A landscape garden is a real luxury to have here in the city.

AH: Agreed, folks of all income and abilities can benefit from herbal gardening, whether you hire someone or do it yourself. What are some of your tricks of the trade?

CW: Dead-head! Constantly! You must dead head your herbs and annuals to keep them beautiful. And if something is looking a little rough midseason, don't be afraid to cut it back and let it re-sprout fresh. Also, I've learned to not be so sentimental. If a plant just isn't working or performing the way you want, sometimes you need to toss it. Never be afraid, even if it's on someone else's dime, to say, "Hey, let's try something else."

AH: Yes, the beauty of growing herbs for use is that when you dead-head to improve productivity and visual appearance, you can use the cuttings medicinally. In landscaping terms, "dead-heading" and "cutting back" are for aesthetic purposes; in medicinal gardening it's called "harvesting!" Can you elaborate on some stories about your work?

CW: Well, in honor of the herbs, I will say that I worked with a very fussy movie star who fancies herself a chef and who asked for a very specific, organically sourced herb and vegetable garden. Not once did the herbs get used! I would go week after week and keep the garden lush and perfect but never did I notice so much of a pinch of parsley missing. So often in my job I think I cater to the dreamy ideas of gardens instead of the use of them. But for me, when I winterized her terrace, I cut it all down and took the biggest bale of fresh herbs home. It was the best Thanksgiving dinner we ever had.

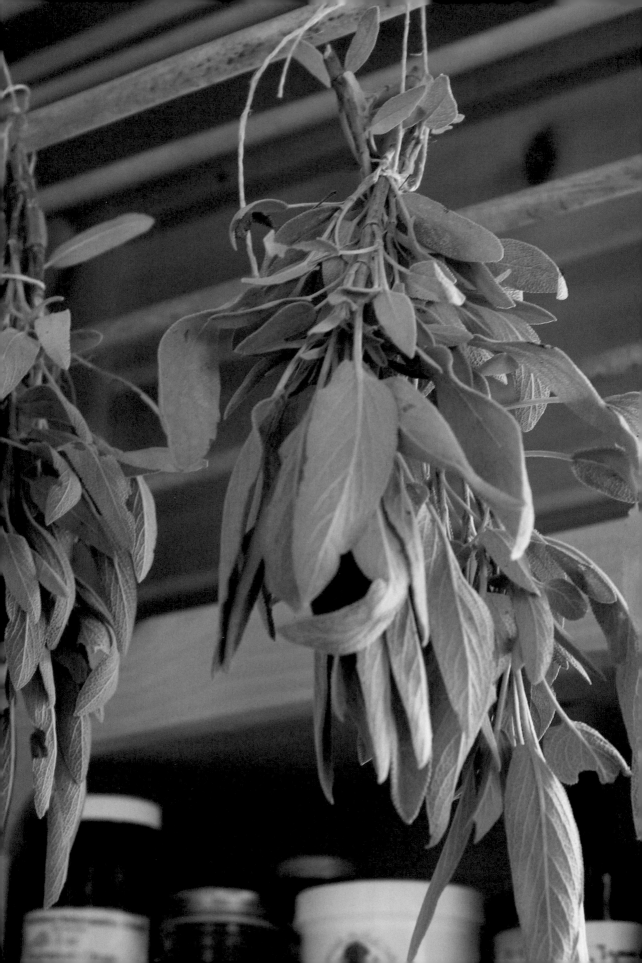

FROM HARVEST TO STORAGE

Don't wait until you're sick to take herbs. The best way to cure illness is not to become ill.

—Rosemary Gladstar,
Family Herbal

Now that you have gotten to know some herbs and have been tending to them, the next step is to integrate them fully into your life for use. This section includes harvesting, processing, and utilizing the herbs you have grown. Drying and storing your herbs for making into medicine in the coming months is a rewarding part of the herbal journey—in a sense to reap what you have sown, and to taste and smell the plants around you in your home throughout the rest of the year.

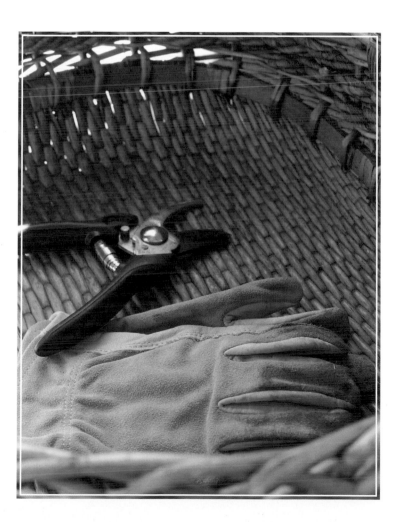

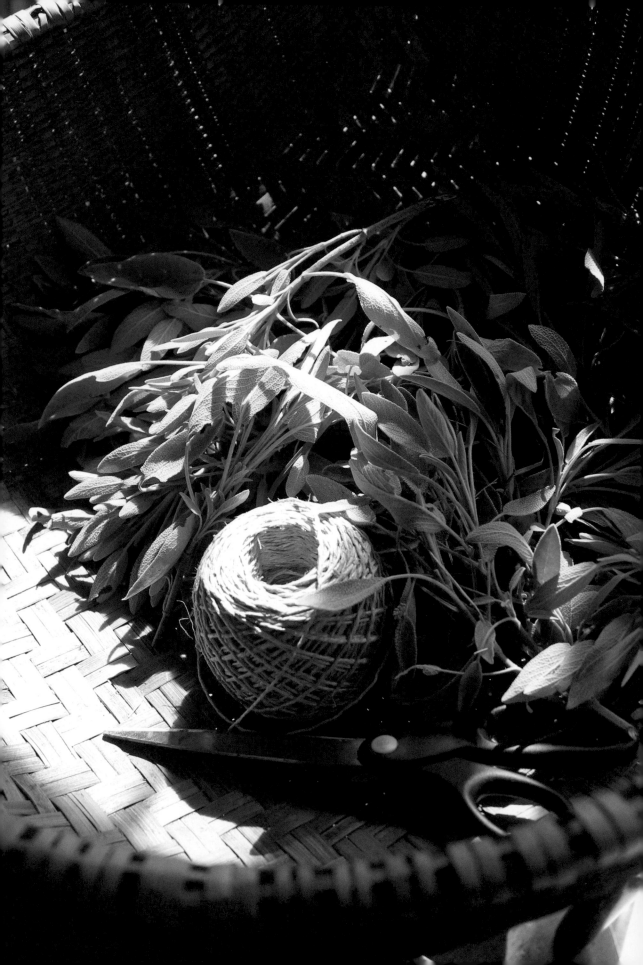

Harvesting

Harvesting depends on the part of the plant that will be used, whether flowers, leaves, roots, bark, or stems. Other factors to plan for in harvesting are time of day and time of year, as this can make a difference in terms of the herbs' ultimate potency and medicinal value.

Harvesting flowers

Flowers are in their prime for picking when they are just at the beginning of the blooming process—just starting to open with all their vitality and sweetness at its peak. This peak time of harvesting will ensure that the plant is putting most of its energy and medicinal properties into the flower at the time of harvest. If the flower is in its fullest bloom with some brown around the edges, it's not the ideal time.

Calendula, elder blossom, and echinacea flowers are a few examples from our "Meet the Plant" list of herbs that have flowers to collect. Elder and echinacea have other parts that can be harvested as well, which we'll cover in the next sections.

After harvesting, the flowers can now be dried or used fresh right away, or put into a menstruum to be extracted. A menstruum is a solvent to extract compounds from plant material. The word *menstruum* originated from the medieval Latin, from "menses," or "month." Oil or alcohol, for example, are mentruums commonly used for the extraction process (see the Simple Home Remedies section).

Harvesting leaves and stems

Herbs that have leaves and stems to be harvested are taken when the plant is putting its energy there. Harvest before the plant has gone to flower, when the buds are just about to open.

Some plants such as nettle—have young shoots in the spring that are packed with nutrients; others, such as Lemon balm or mint, will grow into the season for a little while before maturing to harvest time.

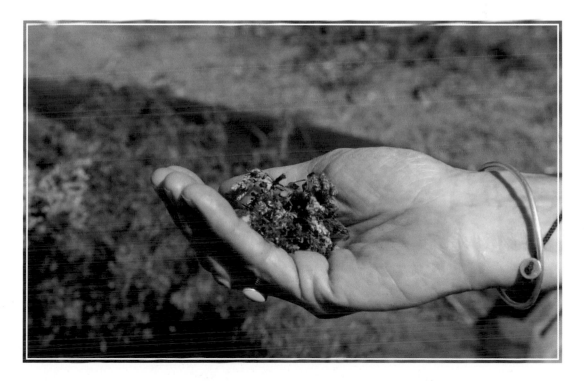

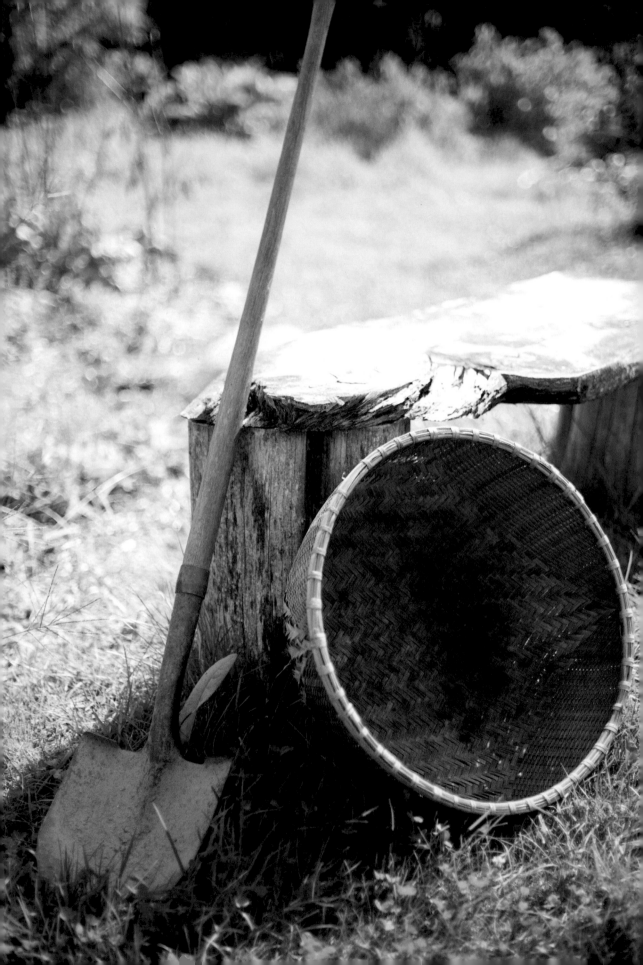

Digging roots

Roots are dug in the spring or fall (preferably fall). Roots are dug only after an herb has been establishing itself in one spot for at least three years (perennials only). In the third year or beyond, harvest some of the roots by gently digging down and separating them out from the others that will be left planted. Disturb as little as possible, and make sure to leave a good amount for the years to come!

While digging up roots for harvest, take some to give away or transplant to another part of your garden if desired. This is the easiest way to propagate perennial herbs—by just separating roots and replanting them.

In the fall plants are sending their energy back down into the earth, and the nutrients and sugars are high in the roots, providing the highest potency for harvesting. Astragalus, echinacea, comfrey, and valerian, to name only a few, are herbs with valuable roots to harvest. Once they are harvested, wash them right away and then chop them. They can then be dried out or placed fresh into an extracting medium (menstruum) such as oil or alcohol for tincture or oil to be strained (decanted) in a few weeks, and used throughout the year (see the Simple Home Remedy section).

Time of year

Generally, leaves are harvested in the spring, and second or third cuttings taken throughout the summer; flowers are cut late spring to early summer, or whenever they are in their prime time of flowering, and roots are cut in the fall, when the energy of growth is going back down into the earth.

Time of day

Herbs like to be harvested in the morning, just when the dew has dried off from the night before, and before the heat of the day sets in. At this time, the herbs are holding the most vibrancy, standing strong and tall.

Tools for harvesting

A sharp harvesting knife (see Resources) or clippers and a basket are the basic tools you will need for harvesting. Gloves may be necessary, depending on your tolerance level, as wild plants usually are the ones with more prickles to defend themselves—such as from nettles, thistles, and raspberry leaves.

Drying

Once you have harvested, there are a few methods for drying on a home scale, and you'll want to proceed with some general rules in mind, and use the most compatible for your current situation.

Drying method #1: The bunch and hang method

For the bunch and hang method, take string and tie up bunches of the herb—not too big or small—and hang in a place where air circulation is good, where not too much direct light will be shining, and where people will not bump into them, or animal hair won't cling. It's important for the bunches to not be too dense in the middle, causing drying of the outside parts and molding of the inside.

Drying method #2: Laying on a screen to dry

Another way to dry fresh cut herbs is to cut up the herb and lay it on a screen or thin cloth, turning periodically. Again,

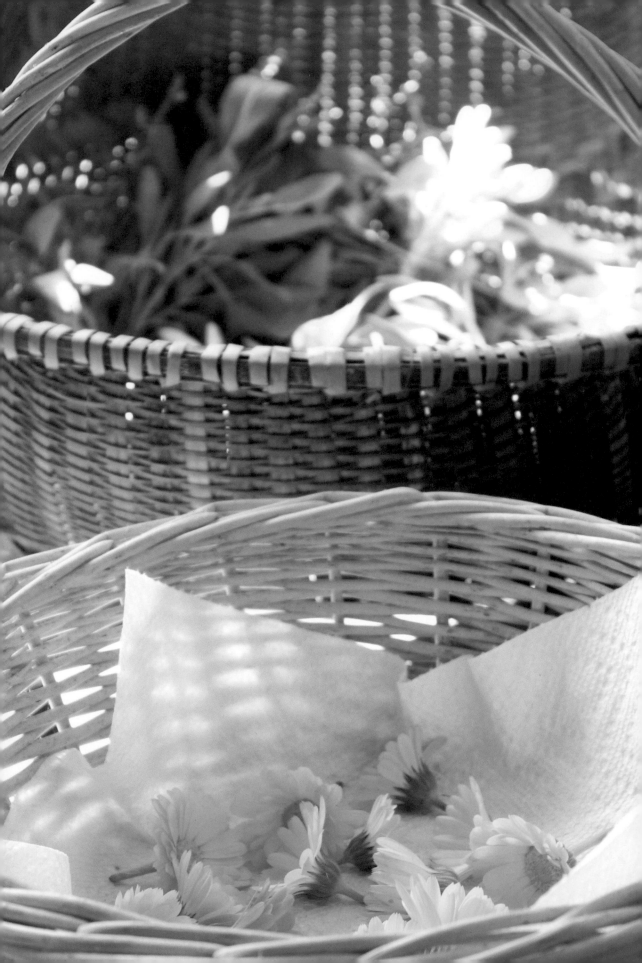

minimal direct light is better, as to not bleach out the properties of the herbs. It's best for herbs to dry out over the course of just a few days, and not be left for too long before being packaged up and stored. They lose their potency when left out too long in the air and light. For instance, if the weather is very humid during the time you are trying to get something dry, try putting a fan on it, and make double sure it is dry all the way through before putting it into a jar or bag. Sometimes if there is a little moisture clinging to the herbs you can transfer the herb to a paper bag for a couple of days where it's still getting air enough to continue drying the last bit but is a little more protected from the light and air, thus curing, and keeping its potency.

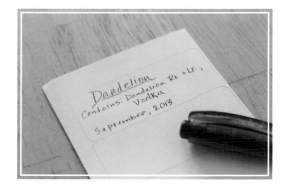

Storage

Once the herbs are totally dry, but not over dried, they are ready for short-/long-term storage. (The way you will know they are dry enough is if the stems are not brittle, yet they are not "elastic" either. Properly dried herbs don't turn into dust when you go to crush them, yet they do not contain moisture.) Glass is preferable overall; plastic can be used for the short term if necessary. Store with a tight fitting lid, away from direct sunlight, and even better, in a cabinet in complete darkness.

Light—any light at all—over time, will deplete the quality of herbs, but in a relatively unlit place, they should be potent for up to a year. Roots will last much longer than leaves and flowers, as the properties are locked in with more density.

Now that your herbs are harvested, you can create your own body care treatments and medicine at home. There are endless opportunities and formulations you can create, which we will talk about in the next section!

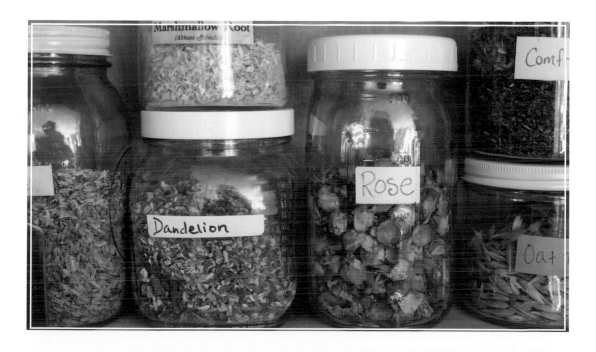

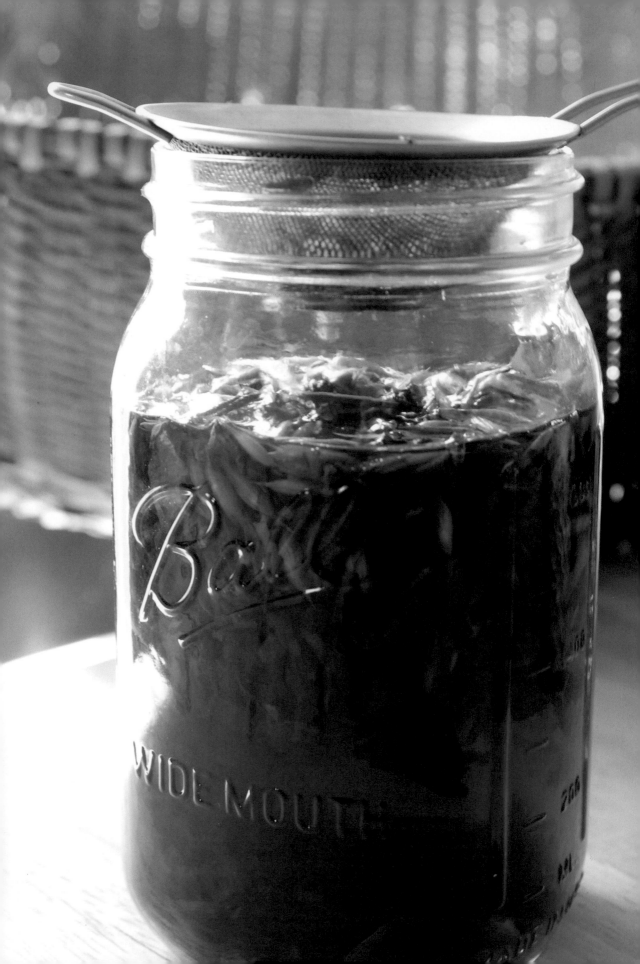

SIMPLE HERBAL MEDICINES & HOME REMEDIES

With the creation of herbal treatments, a relationship as old as the beginning of time is honored and renewed. This relationship with our green friends and the healing gifts they offer to us in the form of herbs, flowers, trees, and fragrances is a relationship offering peace.

—Greta Breedlove, *The Herbal Home Spa*

Fun, creativity, reward, health —after the hard work of growing and gathering, it is time to put our herbs into action. This is our opportunity to be in our kitchens spending time bettering our health, and creating powerful and delicious medicines for our family, friends, and selves.

On the following pages, you will find information, instructions, and recipes that will delight your senses, heal your ailments, and inspire you to further your own experimentation, creativity, and research.

The world is full of methods and recipes for herbal products. Never feel limited. Here we include many ideas for you to build upon.

Herbal infusion

Herbal infusions can be made a few different ways. Tea bags provide convenience when on the go. There are various kinds of contraptions—from tea balls to tea-steeping spoons—that can be used for this process. To get the most out of an herb for pleasure and medicine, the preferred method is working with loose herbs and steeping (which is a more common term for

infusing) for a long period of time; for certain herbs, overnight is best.

Infusions are used for the extraction of vitamins, minerals, and volatile oils, which are naturally occurring delicate oils of the flowers or leaves. The parts of the herbs used are usually the leaves and flowers, opposed to the roots or bark, which are more suitable to a decoction (discussed right after infusions) process.

Instructions for infusion
Fresh Herb Infusion

Take a handful of fresh, chopped herbs, and place it in a quart jar (or use half the amount of herb if you plan on making a pint of infusion). Pour boiling water to fill to the top. Cover and let steep for at least 15 minutes and up to 8 hours. A nice added step here—and with all infusions—would be to place the jar in the sun, for sun tea, or under the moon, for moon tea!

Dry Herb Infusion

If using dry herbs, put about half the amount into the jar, and follow the same instructions.

There are herbs that are great for infusing as simples (by definition one herb), and the combinations of herbs together are endless. Some are better fresh, and some dried. You can make infusions that are highly medicinal, or that are more for taste and pleasure. And they can be beautiful!

Straining

After your herbs have been infused for the requisite amount of time, you can strain the leaves or residue out of the liquid by pouring through a strainer. This process can be made even more enjoyable by choosing or purchasing a strainer that in itself is a beautiful object.

Using

If you are a fan of having your cup of tea hot when you drink it, you can either steep it for a little while, getting partial medicinal value, or you can reheat your infusion that has been steeping for up to 8 hours. You can also add sweetener or juice at any time!

Here are some recipes to play around with. Have fun with this section—mix and match if you so desire—you'll start to feel the benefit of drinking these infusions every day.

Vitamin C Flower Power Blend

1 part rose hips
1 part hibiscus
2 parts lemon balm
1 part dandelion blossoms
½ part roses (whole buds or petals)

This blend will be a vibrant pink, with a very nice flavor, and is great for when you're under the weather or your immunity is low. Rose hips and hibiscus are both loaded with vitamin C, dandelion flowers will help build the blood, and also have many vitamins and nutrients, while the lemon balm is calming to the nervous system, and roses add beauty and flavor.

Super Green Vitamin/Mineral Blend

2 parts nettles
2 parts comfrey
1 part raspberry leaf
1 part yellow dock root
½ part peppermint (optional according to personal taste)

This is a blend that should definitely be steeped for as long as possible, especially because the nettle contains chlorophyll that takes a while to completely release all its goodness. This blend contains the entire spectrum of vitamins and minerals, making it a wonderful medicine for those struggling with low energy. Over time, this blend will build iron levels, help with magnesium and calcium deficiencies, and increase overall strength. Adding a little blackstrap molasses will add some nice sweetness, and more iron richness. The peppermint may not be right for some, and is mostly added to this blend for flavor. Without it, the taste is more earthy and rich.

Relaxation Blend

2 parts chamomile
1 part california poppy
1 part passion flower
½ part lavender
½ part oat tops

This is a beautiful blossom tea to promote relaxation and sleep. Depending on your energy level, this may be a blend to drink throughout the day to ease anxiety, or it may be perfect for the end of a busy day, or for those having trouble sleeping, or who often wake in the night.

Wellness Blend

2 parts astragalus
2 parts elder blossom
2 parts echinacea flowers and/or leaves
1 part tulsi (holy basil)
½ part yarrow
½ part rose hips

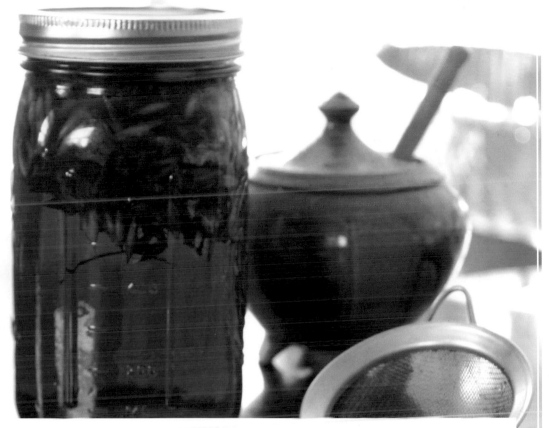

Making Measurements—Simplers Method

There are many ways to measure herbs and other ingredients for the proper formulation of remedies. We choose the Simplers Method—old, folk, simple. It is a combination of art and science, with a lot of room for intuition from you to make a change here and there according to your illness, preference, and liking. This method uses parts, rather than weights or volume. This makes for much flexibility and self-direction in terms of how much you are making. The recipe is laid out in proportion, but the amount that people want to make varies constantly. Whether you'd like to make one pint of infusion, or one quart; four 2-oz. jars of salve, or six—the ratios remain the same, and you figure out the measurements.

We feel that this is the best way to dive in and get the hang of making these medicines firsthand, from your own hand, using your own parts of your own herbs.

Deeply strengthening to the immune system, this blend is helpful when struggling with a cold or flu. It contains vitamin C and many vitamins and minerals that provide a deep immune tonic and stimulating properties. It is slightly diaphoretic, helping the body deal with fever. Add lemon and honey for added benefits and flavor!

Healthy Moon Cycle Blend

2 parts raspberry leaf
1 part nettle
½ part cinnamon
¼ part vitex
¼ part dong quai
¼ part fennel seed
¼ part parsley

A blend for an easeful female cycle, this tea promotes a regular rhythmic cycle, in addition to helping with cramps, and PMS. It's packed with vitamins and minerals for toning the reproductive system and healthy blood.

Energizing Blend

2 parts lemongrass
1 part peppermint
½ part ginseng
½ part eleuthero

This blend is a nice invigorating tea to bring clarity and alertness to one's day. A possible alternative to caffeine, it provides a deep energy, with no crash.

Healthy Gut/Digestion Blend

1 part fennel seed
1 part chamomile
1 part ginger
½ part peppermint
¼ part orange peel

This blend is most effective when drunk along with meals. Stimulates and soothes the digestive tract for all around smoother digestion.

Aphrodisiac Blend

1 part damiana
1 part rose petals
½ part shatavari
½ part orange peel

A mildly euphoric tea, this blend gives an overall feel-good sensation and is wonderful for a date night, or just wanting to feel more loving and open.

Herbal decoction

A decoction is essentially a very strong infusion, made by simmering herbs in water, versus steeping. This strong brew can be used to make syrups, or just consumed straight as potent medicine.

Herbs appropriate for decocting are the tougher, woodier parts of the plants, like roots and bark, and sometimes leaves, but rarely delicate flowers.

Instructions for decoction

On the stovetop, bring 3 parts water and 2 parts fresh herbs, or 1 part dried herbs to a boil. Cover, and let simmer for 15–30 minutes. Remove from heat, let steep for another few minutes, strain, and drink. Or, this decoction can be made into a syrup.

Decoction, unlike infusions, will last in the refrigerator for up to a week.

Some Herbs That Are Great for Decoctions

Burdock Root
Dandelion Root
Astragalus Root
Cinnamon Bark
Marshmallow Root
Echinacea Root
Comfrey Root
Valerian Root
Elder Berries
Hawthorn Berries
Ginger Root
Yellow Dock Root

Syrup

Syrups are a way to make medicine taste great, to prevent spoilage for longer storage, and to get the added medicinal benefits of honey, juices, or molasses. They are usually the preferred way to take medicine for children.

Instructions for Syrup

To make yummy syrup for kids ages 1 and older, follow the instructions for making a decoction (see above), and then add honey, and/or molasses, alcohol, or juice concentrate.

The simplest syrup is one part decoction, one part honey. Mix this combination well and store in the fridge for up to 3 months. You can always add a little alcohol—such as vodka, rum, or brandy—to help preserve it a little more.

For a 4-ounce bottle, add one tablespoon of alcohol.

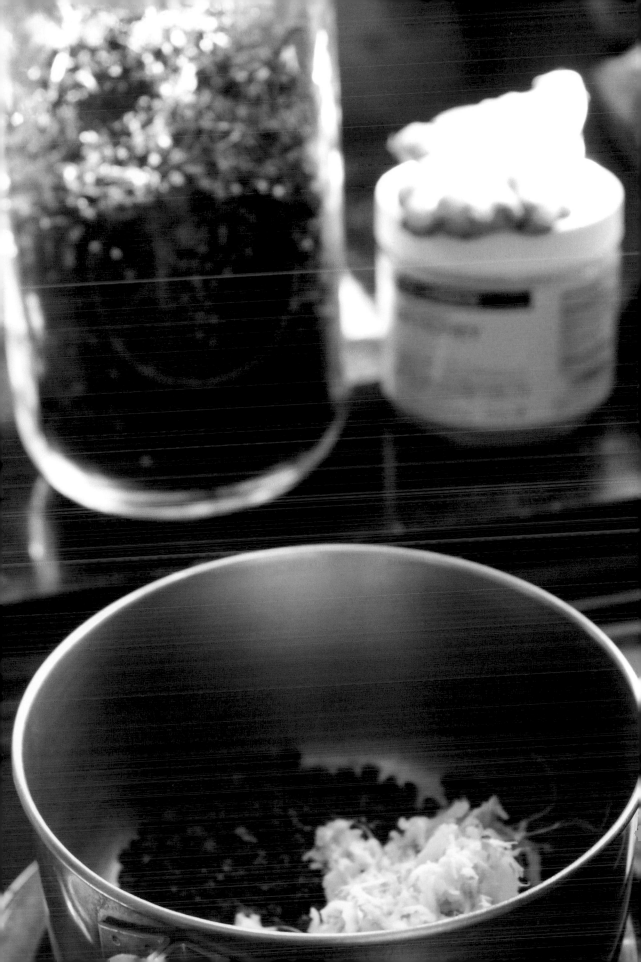

Elderberry Syrup

Follow the directions for making a decoction of elderberries with 1 part ginger root added, fresh or dry.

Strain the herbs out, and measure an equal part honey, while the decoction is still warm. Mix together, pour into your bottle of choice, and store in the fridge.

This is a wonderful medicine for the cold and flu season, both for preventing illness and for relieving acute illness. It will help with viruses of all types, especially in the lungs. The ginger is warming, and helps open the passageways of the body.

Iron and Energy Syrup

2 parts yellow dock
1 part nettle
1 part dandelion root
¼ part kelp
¼ part blackstrap molasses

This is a great syrup to take daily, especially when experiencing low iron levels that lead to fatigue. It's great during pregnancy, when levels are likely to dip down.

Cough Syrup

Make a decoction with the following:
1 part comfrey root
1 part echinacea root
1 part elecampane root
½ part thyme
½ part ginger root
¼ part licorice root

Strain mixture and add an equal part honey, and ½ part black cherry juice.

Mix well, let cool, and store in the fridge.

This formula is ideal for clearing out a wet cough, which tends to want to linger in the winter months!

Stress and Anxiety Support Syrup

Make a decoction with the following:
1 part eleuthero
1 part astragalus

At the end, add the following herbs to steep in the decoction mixture, before straining:
½ part lemon balm
½ part oat tops

Let steep for an hour, strain, and add equal part honey, mix well, let cool, bottle, label, and store in the fridge.

Dental health recipes

Tooth and Gum Health Powder

1 part myrrh gum powder
1 part baking soda
1 part bentonite clay
½ part turmeric powder
½ part slippery elm powder
½ part chamomile powder
¼ part licorice powder
¼ part peppermint powder
¼ part clove powder

This formula is used as toothpaste. Simply dip your damp toothbrush into the powder and brush as usual. It has anti-bacterial, healing, and soothing properties, and it leaves your mouth feeling fresh and clean.

Tooth and Gum Health Mouthwash

1 part comfrey
1 part echinacea
1 part sage
½ part lavender
½ part yarrow

This formula is made as a tincture with the menstruum being equal parts apple cider vinegar and vodka or grain alcohol. After the tincture is finished, it can be bottled in dropper bottles and used as a concentrate. Add one dropper-full to a mouthful of water, and swish for at least 30 seconds.

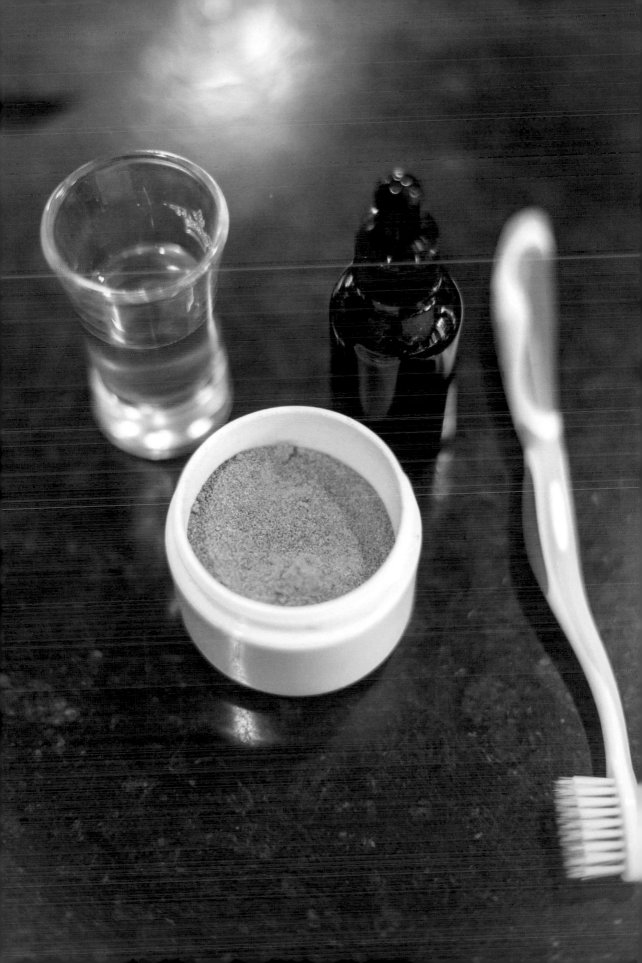

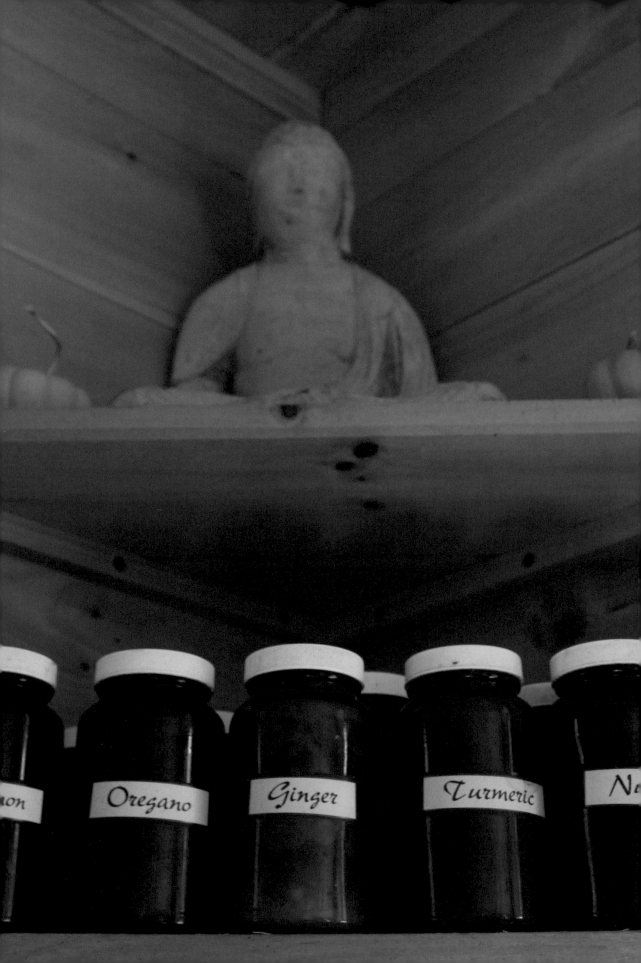

Tincture

Tinctures are alcohol extracts of herbs. Many herbs are well-suited to tincturing, because they have alcohol-soluble components, and some are not.

Tinctures are very easy to make, and are an efficient way to take medicine and have it assimilate into your system quickly. They are great to have with you when traveling, when you cannot brew a cup of tea.

Alcohol goes into your bloodstream immediately and will carry the herbal benefits with it, making tinctures a fast-acting form of herbal medicine.

You can either use fresh or dried herbs, and you can make formulas with more than one herb, or "simples," using only one herb.

Apple cider vinegar or vegetable glycerin can also be used to make tinctures when alcohol is not desired for any reason. Some herbs—such as mineral rich ones—are well suited to vinegar, as the vinegar extracts different components than alcohol. Glycerin is used often for children's formulas for the following reasons: (a) it tastes good, and (b) some parents do not want children ingesting alcohol, even in small quantities.

The Art of Formulation

Creating your own formulas will take time and experience. There is a lot to learn about plants individually, and then how they work with other plants to create a synergy, and therefore, an effective formula. As you go along your journey with herbs, collect as much information as possible on each herb you're getting to know, and eventually you will naturally start to "see" how they can work together— one herb may have a very strong effect, sometimes toxic on its own, but yet after adding a milder, soothing herb, will have an entirely different effect.

In most formulas, there are one or more herbs that are the active herbs—the ones that have the most direct effect on the issue at hand. Then there will be supportive herbs added to those, to round out the formula, and help the more active or stimulating herbs assimilate into the body systems.

In the recipes that follow are some examples of formulas for specific purposes.

Instructions for Tincturing

Fill a jar halfway with dried herbs, or all the way with fresh herbs. Cover completely with menstruum, leaving no air space at the top. Put a lid tightly on the jar, and let sit, shaking daily, for anywhere from 2 to 6 weeks (it won't hurt if it sits longer).

The menstruum is the liquid that will be doing the extraction (i.e., alcohol, alcohol and water, vinegar, or glycerin). Ideally, if you can get hold of a 190-proof organic grain or grape alcohol, use it. In this case you add equal parts distilled, or deep well/clean spring water to it, and that is your menstruum, which you use to cover your herbs for tincturing.

- The other alcohol option is over-the-counter straight 80-proof alcohol. In this case there is no need to add any water, as this is your menstruum. Vodka is most recommended, as it does not impart its own flavor, in turn keeping the medicine more herbal tasting. A lot of liquors have their own attributes that will tend to take over some of the medicinal properties, and override the flavor.
- With vinegar tinctures, use an organic raw apple cider vinegar.
- With glycerin, use organic vegetable glycerin. You can do a combination of this glycerin with alcohol and water as well, if desired.

Once you've had your herb or herbs—whether fresh or dry—and your menstruum co-mingling in a jar together for 2–6 weeks, it's time to reap the benefits! It's time for decanting your medicine.

The next step is to strain out the herbs and pour the tincture into dark bottles for storage and use (see Resources). Using a fine mesh strainer with cheesecloth placed in it, on top of a funnel, pour your mixture through, squeezing all liquid from the plant material. The tincture then can be bottled into smaller dropper-top bottles (see Resources) as needed for use. These bottles are best for being able to get the right dosage (see Appendix 4)

Tincture Recipes

Digestion

2 parts ginger
1 part dandelion root
1 part chamomile
menstruum

Headache

2 parts feverfew
1 part rosemary
1 part lemon balm
½ part lavender
menstruum

Hormonal Balance

2 parts vitex (chaste berry)
1 part red raspberry leaf
1 part wild yam
½ part American ginseng
menstruum

High Mineral Vinegar Tincture

2 parts nettle
1 part horsetail
1 part red raspberry leaf
1 part red clover
1 part cleaned and humanely sourced bones and/or egg shells

Spicy Immunity Vinegar Tincture

1 part ginger—fresh and grated
1 part chili peppers
1 part horseradish—fresh and grated
1 part garlic—fresh, chopped or whole
1 part onions
⅓ part Astragalus
¼ part fresh parsley
½ part honey

Cold and Flu Tincture

2 parts echinacea
2 parts elderberries
1 part goldenseal
1 part boneset
½ part ginger
½ part thyme
¼ part garlic
¼ part raw, local honey

This formula is indicated when strong cold and/or flu symptoms are present, such as fever, body aches, lots of congestion, intense sore throat, and cough.

Kids Calming Glycerite

1 part lemon balm
1 part chamomile
1 part tulsi basil
½ part valerian

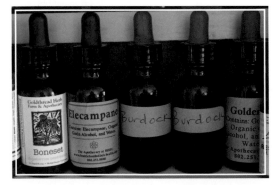

Powdered herbs

Powdered herbs come in handy for a few different preparations including capsules, pill balls, and poultices.

You can make your own herbs into powders at home with a good quality herb grinder or a coffee grinder. You can also—of course—order them from an herb company (see Resources).

Once you have the powders you'd like to work with, they can be stored in an airtight container—preferably glass, away from light—for some time, up to 6 months at the most, for potency sake.

Instructions for capsules

You'll want to buy a hand encapsulater (see Resources). These are great little tools that make it easy to make 24 capsules at one time, instead of packing each empty capsule separately—so tedious!

You will also need to purchase empty capsules (see Resources). There are a couple of different types and sizes. Make sure the encapsulator size matches the capsule size you are using.

Follow directions for use, and start making capsules for you and your friends and family! This is a nice way to take medicine on the go (they store well), and some herbs, well, you just don't want to have to taste. (See Appendix 4 for dosage recommendations.)

Herbal Capsule Recipes

Stomach Ease

2 parts ginger
1 part slippery elm
1 part chamomile
½ part fennel

Beautiful Skin

1 part dandelion root
1 part nettle
1 part yellow dock
½ part red clover

Cold Care

2 parts echinacea root
2 parts astragalus
1 part ginger
½ part goldenseal
½ part myrrh

Another way to incorporate herbal powders into your medicine chest are pill balls—these are fun, can taste great, and can be a nice way to entice children to take herbs. Basically, you are just making dough with the powders and a few other ingredients, such as honey or nut butters mixed in. Getting the desired consistency is an art, not a science, so play around here! You can make them as big or small as you'd like, they can even be a substantial snack for small and large children alike.

Instructions for herbal pill balls

This is pretty free form. Once you have powdered the herbs you'd like to incorporate, just play around with amounts, and other ingredients, until you have the desired consistency and flavors. You really cannot go wrong.

Some ingredients to incorporate into pill balls besides the herbs:
nut butters
honey
ghee (clarified butter)
dates, and other dried fruits
coconut flour, oil, or shredded meat
sesame, poppy, or flax seeds

Recipes for Herbal Pill Balls

Immunity Balls

3 parts astragalus
1 part echinacea
½ part dandelion
½ part lemon balm

Energy Balls

2 parts gaurana
1 part carob
1 part cacao
½ part mint

Spice Balls

1 part turmeric
1 part ginger
½ part cinnamon
¼ part cloves

Poultice

A poultice is one of the simplest and quickest ways to administer herbal medicine topically. In a sense you literally can grab it out of the ground and put it on you! It is most likely the oldest form of herbal medicine.

A poultice is the application of fresh or dried powdered herbs and hot or warm water.

Poultice Uses

heal wounds
soothe rashes
draw out splinters
heal bee stings and bug bites
reduce enlarged glands
bring boils to a head
ease acne
cool inflammation
help joint pain
ease headaches
shrink tumors and cysts

Instructions for Making a Poultice

Measure the desired amount of herbal powder—enough for the area that you will be immediately using it for (i.e., a small amount)—and mix with enough water to make a nice paste, not too runny or chunky. The temperature of the poultice when applied will need to be hot if you need to draw something to a head, and only warm if you want a soothing effect.

Once the paste is made, you can apply it directly on the area in need, or put the paste into a muslin cloth (like cheesecloth), then apply that to the skin. This way makes less mess!

Now, for best results and to retain the heat of the poultice, apply another warm moist cloth over it, and even a layer of plastic wrap. To ensure even longer-term heat and effectiveness, place a hot water bottle or hot pack over the whole thing. Now rest; let the poultice penetrate and heal, unwrap, repeat if necessary.

For quick first-aid situations, such as a bee sting, it is effective to just pick a fresh herb from the yard, crush it up—even chew it up—and apply it immediately. Try to hold it on the sting, after pulling the stinger out, for a little while

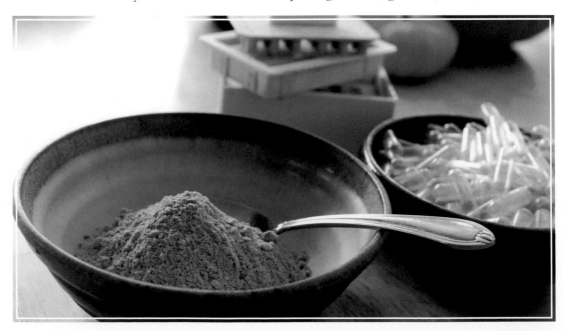

until the pain and swelling subside. This is very effective for children when they are in the throes of the pain. Also, more casual ways, like just putting clay paste onto poison ivy and letting it dry out to draw the pus, can work wonders!

Poultice Recipes

Plantain

Plantain is amazing at immediately bringing down inflammation in a sting or bite and easing the pain. Luckily this plant is everywhere we step, growing in our lawns, and often as a wonderful weed in the garden. You can either just pick a leaf, chew it up into a pulp, apply, press, and wrap, or mix with hot water and use any or all of the previous techniques for application.

Plantain is one of the best first-aid remedies.

Sage

Use sage powder or the fresh herb, crushed.

Add hot water to make the desired consistency.

A poultice of sage is very astringent, and will draw out splinters, pus, and generally heal the area.

Mustard

Use mustard powder. Add hot water to make the desired consistency.

Mustard is an age-old remedy for sore muscles, sore throat, and enlarged lymph glands.

Follow the instructions above, making sure to put the mustard paste into cloth before applying, because it can burn or irritate the skin if put directly on it.

Yarrow

Mash up fresh yarrow with some warm water—or saliva—and place directly on a wound.

This is an antiseptic first aid to stop bleeding as well as keep out/clean out bacteria that may have entered the wound.

Herbal oils

Herbal oils are made by a simple process of infusing an herb or herbs into a carrier oil (i.e., olive, almond, coconut, jojoba). They can be highly medicinal for first-aid situations, or they can be luxurious body oils.

Herbal oils can then be used to make a salve, ointment, body butter, or lip balm; or they can be used as is, and you can choose essential oils to add for aromatherapy and medicinal value.

Herbal oils can be made with fresh herbs, slightly dried herbs, or fully dried herbs. The ratios will vary accordingly.

Instructions for Herbal Oils

Take 1 part dried herb to 2 parts oil of choice (see carrier oil list that follows). Put into a jar, and let sit in a sunny spot for 2–4 weeks, shaking daily. If using fresh or slightly dried herbs, fill the jar with the herb, and cover with oil.

Always make sure that the oil is covering the herbs, and filled all the way to the top of whatever jar you are using—this will make oxidation and mold on the top of the oil less likely. If using fresh herbs, there is more likeliness for mold to occur, as the herbs still contain water. Check daily for mold, and scrape off any, and smell to make sure all is well. Fresh herbal oils are more potent than dried.

TIP: One method to lessen the likeliness for mold is to "wilt" the herbs overnight, to get out some of the water, but still have them be mostly fresh.

After 2–4 weeks, your oil is ready for decantation (straining and bottling, or using to make another remedy). Simply strain through a mesh strainer with cheese-cloth laid in it, making sure the oil comes through clear. This is now the time to add essential oils if desired—you can play around with the amount, to your liking. In general, about 15 drops per one ounce of oil. (See the list below of essential oils.)

Stovetop Herbal Oil Instructions

In a double boiler, heat appropriate amounts of desired herbs and oils together, and simmer over low heat stirring occasionally for about an hour. Strain, let cool completely. This is a quick and convenient way to infuse an herbal oil, but not quite as effective as infusing over time in a warm spot and shaking daily.

Bottle into dark bottles—amber, blue, green, etc. (see Resources)—label and store!

Some Carrier Oils and Their Benefits

Coconut—emollient, conditioning, protecting

Olive—emollient, restorative

Jojoba—emollient, antioxidant

Sweet almond—emollient, fragrant

Apricot kernel—emollient, fragrant, used for massage

Sesame—emollient, UV protection, mildly cleansing

Grape-seed—emollient, non-allergenic, non-greasy

Some Essential Oils and Their Benefits

Lavender—relaxing, soothing

Sage—antibacterial, cleansing

Lemon—uplifting

Eucalyptus—invigorating, clears passage-ways

Rose—amazing for skin rejuvenation, oils contained in roses are similar in substance to skins own oils—making them easily absorbed and utilized.

Lemon grass—uplifting

Peppermint—rejuvenating

Herbal Oil Recipes

Trauma Oil

equal parts St. John's wort, arnica, and calendula

olive oil (enough to cover herbs)

The synergy of St. John's wort, arnica, and calendula working together is close to miraculous! This oil can be applied topically when there is injurious trauma (not to be applied to open skin), or to heal bruises rapidly. It penetrates deeply, and often provides immediate relief.

A couple of years ago I was gathering firewood. I was getting tired and had a few more pieces to split to be finished for the day. I was working with black birch, which can have twisted grain requiring a lot of force to split. This particular piece was about 18 inches long and I had a split started and then turned it a quarter turn hoping that when I hit it with all my might it would break into four pieces. I raised the ax and with all the power I had, I brought the ax down on the wood. It did come apart with a lot of force and one piece shot into my right shin. I went white with pain. Another piece slid up the handle of the axe and tore off half of my knuckle on the index finger of my right hand. My finger started bleeding profusely from under the flap of skin. I didn't even notice the pain of my finger because my shin was throbbing and swollen. I was on the ground writhing, unable to stand up. Alyssa heard the commotion and came to see what had happened. She immediately ran back into our yurt and grabbed some trauma oil and cayenne pepper. She started rubbing my shin with the oil and within 5 seconds the pain had all but vanished and I could stand up. I couldn't believe how quickly it brought relief! That gave me enough breathing room to look at my finger, which was still bleeding. Alyssa put some cayenne pepper in the wound to stop the bleeding, which it did. Five stitches later and with regular doses of trauma oil it was as if it had never happened. I have had many healing experiences with herbs but that was amazing. I carry trauma oil with me all the time now in my first-aid medicine bag.

—Bret Holmes

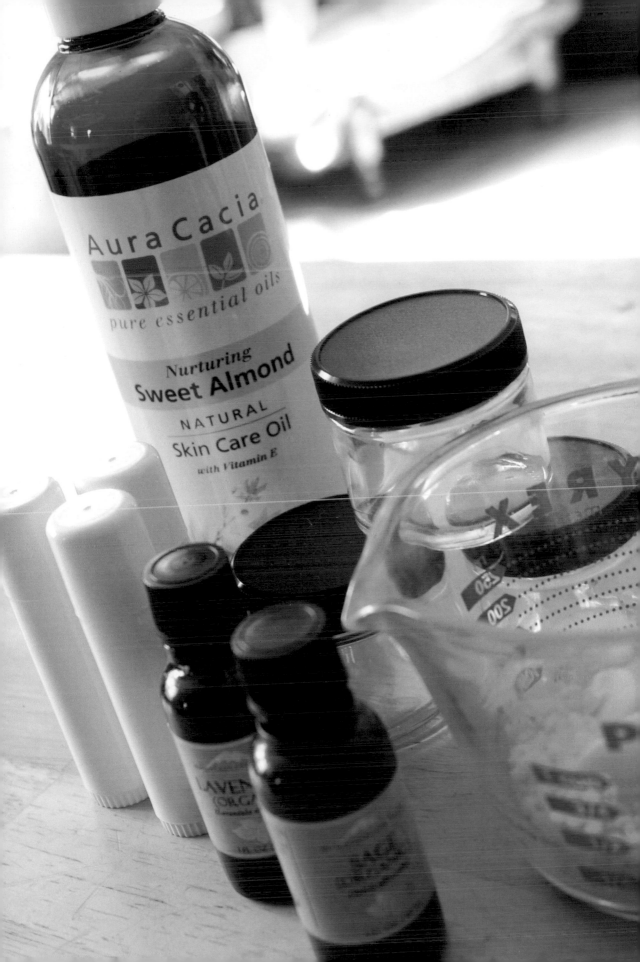

Beautiful Body Oil

Equal parts calendula, rose, and chamomile
2 parts olive oil
1 part sweet almond oil
½ part coconut oil
½ part jojoba oil
Essential oils of lavender, lemon grass, and sage (about 15 drops essential oil total per ounce of herbal oil)

Skin Healing Oil

2 parts comfrey leaf
1 part calendula
1 part elder flowers
1 part plantain
2 parts olive oil
½ part coconut oil

Sunshine Oil

1 part St. John's wort–infused olive oil
1 part cold-pressed, unrefined coconut oil
lavender essential oil if desired

This oil can be applied either before, while in, or after being in the sun. It helps our skin assimilate the vitamin D and the healthy aspects of the sun into our bodies—which is so essential for overall health.

Salve, body butter, and lip balm

A salve is a medicinal preparation for topical use, prepared by thickening an herbal oil (see the previous section on herbal oils) with wax, generally beeswax.

Body butters and lip balm have more ingredients—namely butters—added in to make a creamier consistency. Shea butter and coco a butter are examples.

Essential oils and liquid vitamins can be added for medicinal, aromatherapy, and preservation purposes.

Salves are useful in so many situations including skin infections, scrapes and bruises, diaper rash, eczema, chicken pox, poison ivy, and dry skin. They are applied to skin that is not open or oozing, and sometimes to a wound that is inflamed and in danger of infection.

Salves, body butter, and lip balms are easy to store, carry, and use as they are a bit less messy than a straight herbal oil. All preparations have their appropriate time and place. They also make great gifts!

Instructions for Salve, Body Butter, and Lip Balm

Start by measuring the right amounts of herbal oil and beeswax. The general ratio here for salve is 4 parts oil to 1 part wax. If you are also adding butter(s), depending on the consistency you want, add a little less wax. The way to test the consistency is to dip a spoon into the mixture as it is melting on the stovetop, let it harden, then try it out. You can then add more oil if too hard, or more wax and/or butters, if too soft.

Beeswax can be challenging to chop and measure—here are some ideas to make it easier!

If you are working with a chunk or chunks of wax, just wrap it in cloth and pound with a hammer until it is broken up into workable pieces. The smaller the pieces, the easier it is to measure. Fortunately, there is beeswax available on the market now that is already broken into tiny "pearls" that is so incredibly nice to work with (see Resources).

Next, get a double boiler going on the stove, and add the herbal oil and wax and/or butters. Let them melt together, and stir once just to make sure they are very well mixed. Turn the heat off, remove the top of the double boiler with your mixture in it, let cool just a bit, and add essential oils or vitamins at this time.

Before the mixture is cooled enough to begin hardening in the pot, pour into the containers. Dark containers are ideal for longer-term storage. But any container with a wide mouth (for salves and butters) will do, and smaller tins or lip balm tubes for lip balm (see Resources).

Let cool completely before putting on the covers. Label and you're done!

Recipes for salves, body butters, and lip balms

Antibacterial Salve

4 parts herbal oil made with olive oil infused with:
  1 part goldenseal
  1 part echinacea root
  1 part myrrh gum
1 part beeswax
10 drops pure vitamin E oil per 1 ounce of salve

Soothing, Healing Body Butter

4 parts herbal oil made with sweet almond oil infused with:
  2 parts calendula
  1 part comfrey
  1 part plantain

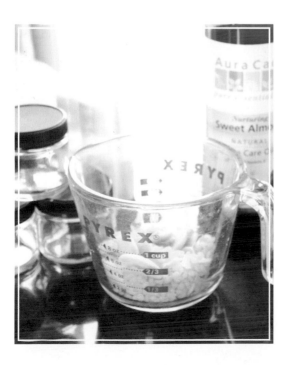

½ part beeswax
1 part cocoa butter
15 drops lavender essential oil per 1 ounce body butter

Shea Vanilla Lip Balm

4 parts herbal oil made with apricot kernel oil infused with calendula
1 part beeswax
1–2 parts shea butter—it will need to be a harder consistency if going into lip balm tubes than it will if going into tins. Test a small batch to get the desired consistency.
15 drops of vanilla essential oil per 1 ounce of lip balm

Liniment

An herbal liniment is used as a disinfectant for wounds, or as a rub for sore muscles. It is made exactly like a tincture, except the menstruum is either witch hazel or rubbing alcohol. The ratio of herb to liquid is the same, and the time it takes to macerate is the same. (See the Tincture section.)

Liniments are quite powerful and are for external use only. They can have miraculous cleansing abilities with stubborn, festering wounds, while also aiding in the healing process! They are often used in massage for muscle aches, pain, and inflammation, especially in Asia. One more use is for headaches—you can rub them on the temples, or wherever it hurts on the head, and often this will extract some, if not all, of the pain.

Make sure to wash hands after use, avoid eyes, and keep out of reach from children.

Kloss's Liniment Recipe

This is a famous recipe from Dr. Jethro Kloss (*Back to Eden*)

1 ounce echinacea powder
1 ounce goldenseal powder

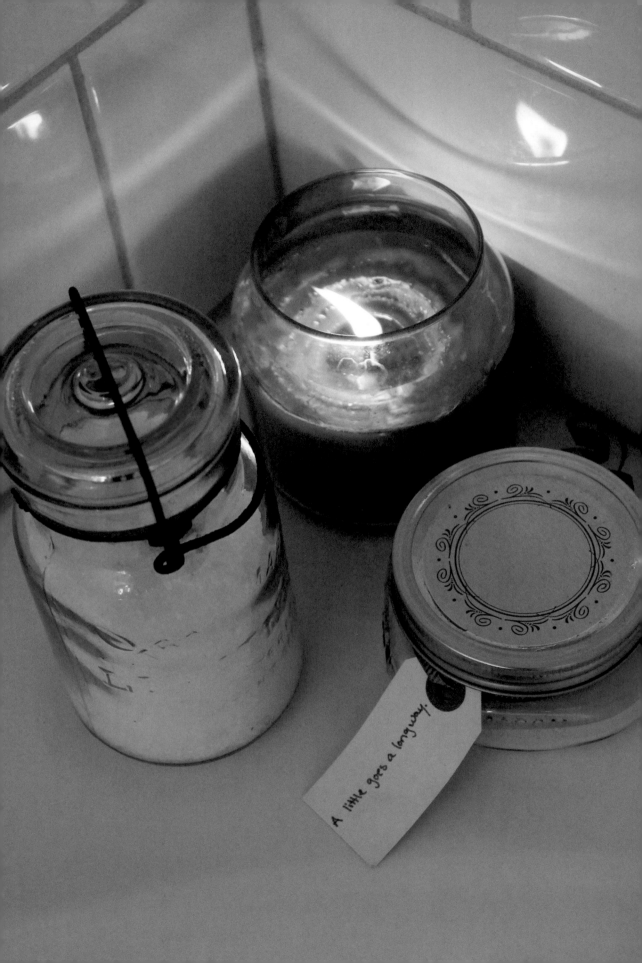

A little goes a long way.

1 ounce myrrh powder
¼ ounce cayenne powder
1 pint rubbing alcohol

Kloss liniment is effective against wounds and sore inflamed muscles. It's an incredible medicine to have on hand for first aid.

Herbal baths

An herbal bath can often be just the answer we are looking for to calm nerves and relieve stress. Our skin, being the body's largest organ, will drink in the contents of what we put into the bath. There is so much opportunity for healing in the water, whether hot, tepid, or cold. Candles can help relieve stress, too.

In the bath, we can ease poison ivy; soothe sore, overused muscles; detoxify our systems; heal scratched and bug-bitten skin; and re-center ourselves to emerge anew.

Instructions for an Herbal Bath

Method 1: In a large soup pot on the stove heat 1 or 2 gallons of water to a boil. Add 3 large handfuls of herbs, dried or fresh. Remove from heat, cover, and let mixture steep for anywhere from 10 minutes to an hour. Strain out herbs, and add this tea to your bathwater.

Method 2: Fill a sachet—a muslin bag with a tie—with herbs, and tie it to the faucet, as you run the hot water for the bath. The water will run through it, and make tea as it goes. Or, you can just add the bag of herbs directly into the bathtub. With this method, you can then use the "tea bag" to massage your body with.

By bathing, you are drinking the herbal infusion through your skin. The hotter the water, the more open your pores will be, therefore the more you will drink in. Cooler water is more toning and strengthening to the body,

and can be used to bring down fevers slightly, and to tone and strengthen the skin and organs.

Recipes for Herbal Baths

Relaxation

1 cup of salts (i.e., sea, epsom, pink, etc.)
1 cup of baking soda
1 cup chamomile
1 cup lavender
1 cup hops
20 drops lavender essential oil

Cold and Flu

1 cup equal parts epsom and sea salt
1 cup baking soda
1 cup yarrow
1 cup elder flowers
1 cup chamomile
30 drops eucalyptus essential oil

Lavender Oatmeal for Itchy Skin

2 cups ground dry rolled oats
1 cup salts of choice
30 drops lavender essential oil

Healing After Birth Sitz Bath

1 part yarrow
1 part comfrey
1 part calendula
1 part plantain
½ part sage
sea salt and/or Epsom salt if desired

When you are ready to take a bath (most likely a few days after giving birth), making a tea from this formula and adding it to a shallow bath is super healing for all the tissues down there. Soak for twenty minutes, and repeat daily if necessary.

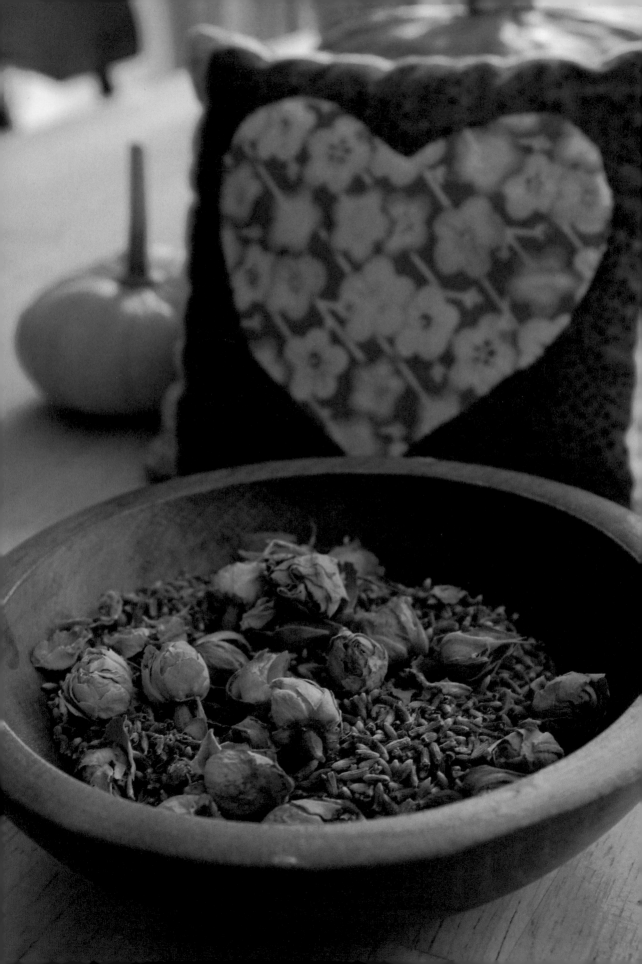

Benefits of salts and baking soda

- Epsom salts—soothe sore muscles and add magnesium through the skin to help with leg cramps, dry skin, and general magnesium deficiency
- Dead sea salts—full of minerals and trace minerals
- Sea salt—skin soothing, full of minerals
- Baking soda—soothing, softening effect, great for skin and muscles, neutralizes chlorine

Sachets and Dream pillows

Sachets and dream pillows are the same thing, each having its own purpose. A sachet can be used to put in drawers of clothing to keep bugs out and make clothes smell nice or can be hung in your car instead of the smelly cardboard trees from the convenience store! They make nice gifts, and when the herbs lose potency after a while, they can be opened up and new herbs added.

A dream pillow is used to enhance dreaming and relaxation. It is a fine companion to take to bed, ensuring comfort and sleepy bliss.

Instructions for sachet and dream pillow

Method for Sachet

Simply take a square piece of cloth that is thin, and about 1 foot. Lay on a flat surface, and place 1 or 2 cups of nice smelling dried herbs of choice into the middle. Scoop up all the edges, wrapping the herbs in the middle, and tie a string or ribbon around it tight. Voila—simple as that! It's nice to use beautiful material and string—be creative.

Method for Dream Pillow

Here is where a little sewing comes in to play. Choose material that is thin enoughso that you can smell the herbs through it, of course. Sew—either by hand or machine—a pillow in the shape of your choice. When it is nearly fully sewn, fill up with herbs, and sew up the hole. There is the option of adding other ingredients to the pillow to add texture and/or density; such as: buckwheat hulls, rice, or dry beans.

Recipe for Sachet

2 parts lavender
2 parts roses
1 part lemon balm or lemongrass
½ part mint

Recipe for Dream Pillow

2 parts mugwort
1 part lavender
1 part chamomile
1 part hops

Smudges and Smudging

Burning herbs is a sacred practice used for purification and prayer in many Native American traditions. Sage is a very common herb used for smudging (burning). Sage is a purifier—it cleanses an area, sweeping away negativity. This practice is often used in a sacred circle setting, like a birth circle, or to purify a space where there may be negative energy or spirits.

You can just burn small pieces of dried sage in a flameproof vessel, or you can make a smudge stick.

Smudge stick

To make a smudge stick, take several stalks of fresh sage, and bind them together lengthwise by wrapping string—hemp preferred—around them, spiraling down the whole thing to create a "wand." Let sit in a warm dry place for several days to cure and dry. *(continued)*

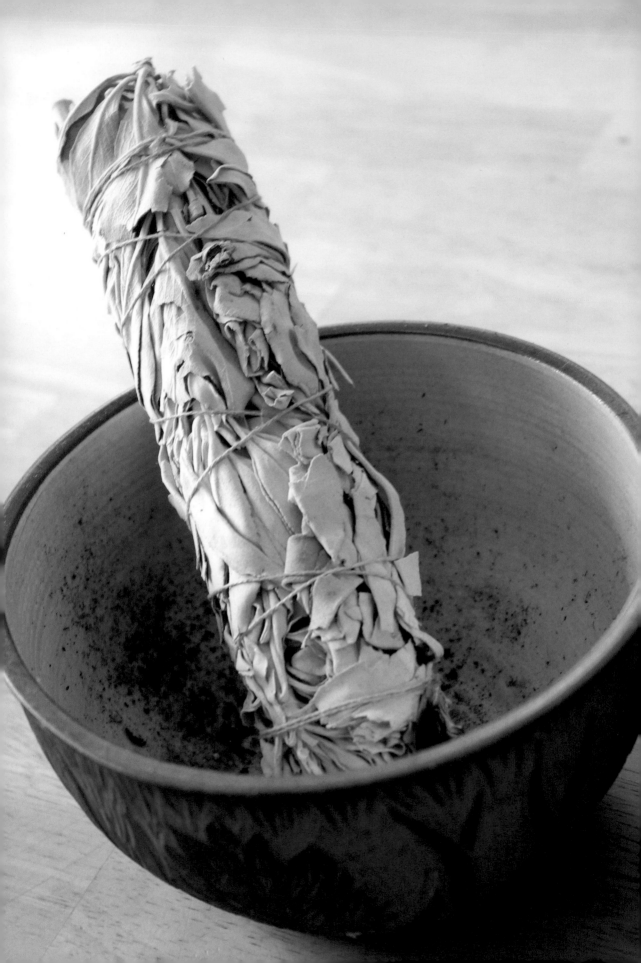

Light the tip of it when ready to smudge, and it should smoke nicely. When done smudging, make sure to tamp it out, so there are no embers remaining, and store it in a fireproof container.

For more recipes, ideas, and suggestions—specifically related to immune health and diseases of the gut, see Appendix 2.

Go forth into the unlimited world of medicine making, where science meets magic, and we infuse ourselves with the plants and become one with this ancient craft!

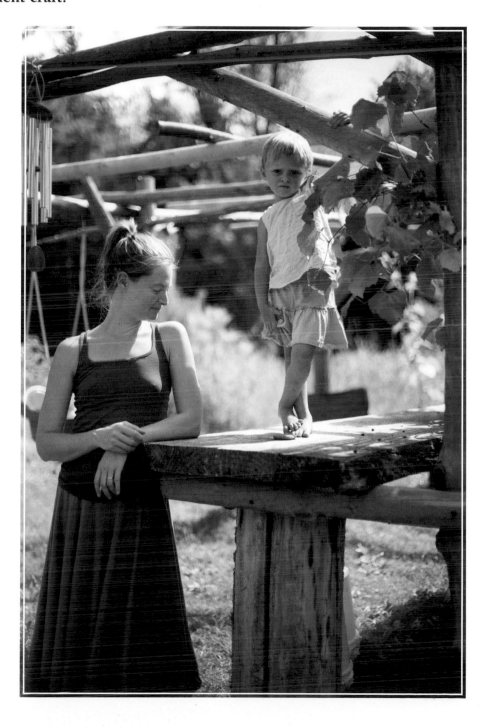

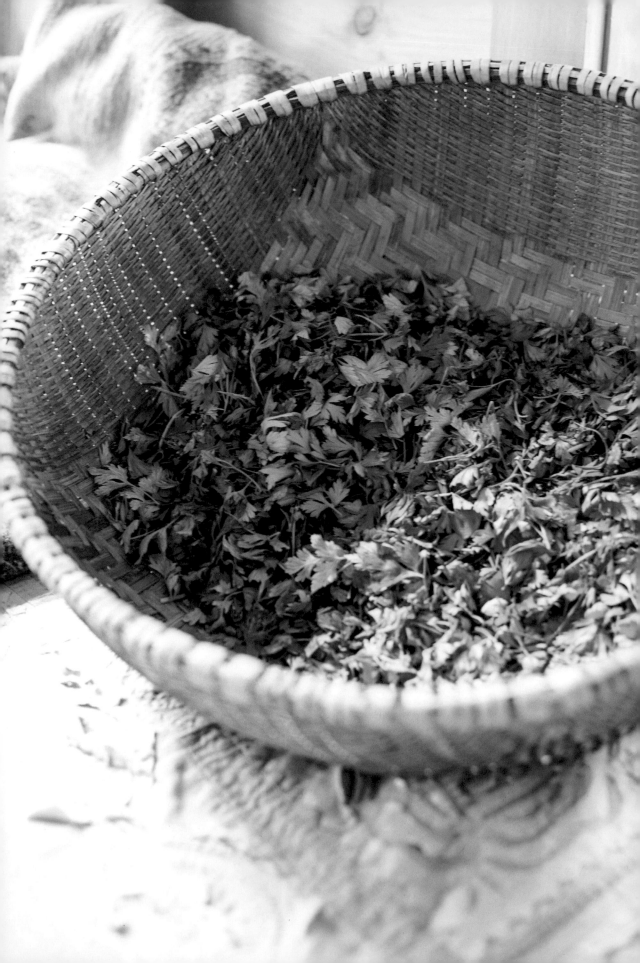

CONCLUSION

We humans want connection. It is vital for us to feel loved and cared for, nourished and healthy, and when we are feeling these things, we feel connected; connected with our bodies, other people, the environment that surrounds us, and the earth. Being connected with our well-being, with what makes us feel healthy and whole, is important for a long, fulfilled life.

Getting to know and be able to use some medicinal plants is a very direct and rewarding way to experience connection. They very quickly connect us with the earth from where they come, as well as connecting us to the rich history and traditions of their uses. And very importantly, they connect us with our bodies—by working with our systems to treat, balance, tonify, and nourish.

It can be so exciting to ignite the flame of inner and outer health and radiance! To create or continue a connection with the earth and our health in this way —with the herbs. Herbs truly are our allies in this life, especially in this time of toxicity in our water, food, and air. As a whole people, we are craving optimum health, simplicity, connection.

Planting a garden of whatever type, whether big or small, gets us in touch with the elements, the earth. Getting out in the sunshine and in the rain, in itself is healing. Growing some herbs, bringing them into your home, processing them, and transforming them into medicine or body care is a simple practice that improves your overall sense of well-being, and can instill confidence in your ability to heal and help others.

We hope this book has given you tools to be a grower of plants, a healer of wounds . . . an herbalist. We hope that it kindles a deeper connection with this ancient practice, and that you and your family and friends can benefit from the plants themselves in your garden, and the wonderful medicines you have in your home.

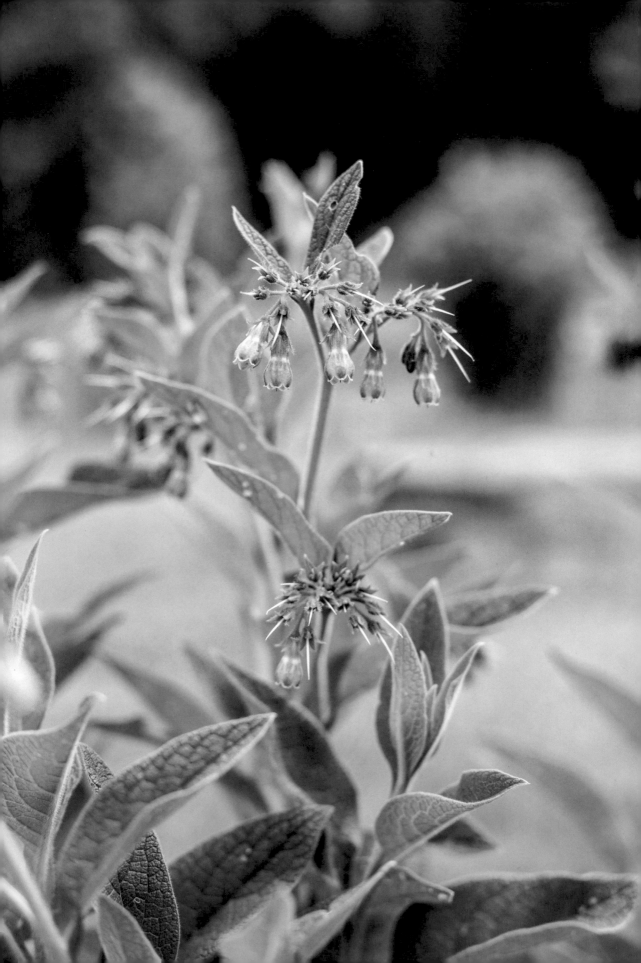

APPENDIX 1

Properties and Actions of Herbs

Included here are descriptions of some of the many properties and actions of herbs, with examples of specific herbs to follow.

Abortifacient: Can cause expulsion of the fetus, and if not, can cause other damage to fetus.
Blue cohosh, mugwort, pennyroyal.

Adaptogen: Helps our body adapt to and deal with stress in all areas— body, mind, spirit. Helps keep balance and conserve energy.
Astragalus, ashwaganda, ginseng, eleuthero.

Alterative: Blood purifiers, cleansers, builders, tonics. Helps the body deal with toxic substances, and to assimilate nutrients.
Burdock, comfrey, nettle, plantain.

Analgesic: Relieves pain.
Chamomile, skullcap, valerian.

Anodyne: Relieves pain (see Analgesic).

Antiarthritic: Relieves inflammation and joint pain. Protects joints from degeneration.
Turmeric, juniper, black cohosh.

Antibacterial: Inhibits the growth of, or destroys bacteria and viruses.
Echinacea, elecampane, garlic, goldenseal.

Anticatarrhal: Decreases mucous production.
Elder, mullein, sage.

Antipyretic: Cooling to reduce or prevent fever.
Boneset, basil, chickweed.

Antidepressant: Relieves depression, supports the nervous system.
Lemon balm, oat tops, St. John's wort.

Antiemetic: Prevents vomiting.
Chamomile, ginger, peppermint.

Antifungal: Inhibits or destroys growth of fungi.
Garlic, tea tree, yarrow.

Anti-inflammatory: Reduces inflammation.
Cayenne, chamomile, turmeric, yarrow.

Antilithic: Prevents kidney stones.
Corn silk, gravel root, hydrangea.

Antimicrobial: Reduces microbial growth, same as antibacterial.

Antioxidant: Prevents damage from free radicals.
Astragalus, ginger, sage, turmeric.

Antiparasitic: kills parasites. Not to be used in excess.
Clove, elecampane, wormwood, garlic.

Antiseptic: Cleansing to the skin topically to prevent microbes and infection.
Calendula, sage, plantain, yarrow.

Antispasmodic: reduces muscle spasm, relaxes muscles.
Chamomile, cramp bark, kava, valerian.

Antitussive: Relieves coughing.
Elecampane, coltsfoot, poppy, thyme.

Antitumor: Suppresses growth of tumors.
Astragalus, burdock, echinacea, garlic, red clover.

Antiviral: Supports the immune system and suppresses the growth of viruses.
Elder, lemon balm, garlic, echinacea, osha.

Aphrodisiac: Tones reproductive organs, and/or stimulates sexual desire.
Astragalus, ginseng, damiana, burdock.

Astringent: Constricting of tissues, used to bind swellings, bleeding, and mucous membranes.
Mullein, red raspberry, sage, yarrow.

Bitter: Stimulates digestion, by increasing production of bile.
Burdock, dandelion, motherwort, yarrow.

Bronchodilator: Relaxes bronchial muscles, to create easier breathing.
Chamomile, elecampane, peppermint, thyme.

Calmative: Calming to the nervous system.
Chamomile, hops, lavender, valerian.

Carminative: Relieves gas and griping. Fennel, ginger, peppermint.

Cholagogue: Promotes bile flow from the gall bladder. These herbs also have laxative properties. Burdock, dandelion, goldenseal.

Choleretic: Stimulates bile production in the liver. (See Bitter and Cholagogue herbs).

Demulcent: Soothes and heals mucous membranes. Marshmallow, comfrey, slippery elm, burdock, fenugreek.

Diaphoretic: Induces sweating. Elder, peppermint, yarrow.

Diuretic: increases and stimulates urination. Burdock, dandelion, elder, nettle, parsley.

Emmenagogue: Stimulates suppressed menstruation. Blue cohosh, pennyroyal, yarrow.

Emetic: Induces vomiting. Bloodroot, ipecac, lobelia.

Emollient: Protects, soothes and softens the skin. Oils of almond, apricot, sesame, and olive. Comfrey root, slippery elm, chickweed.

Expectorant: Expels mucous. Comfrey, elecampane, coltsfoot, mullein, horehound.

Galactagogue: Increases milk flow. Blessed thistle, fennel, dandelion, alfalfa, oat tops.

Heart tonic: Supports and strengthens natural functions of the heart. Hawthorne, motherwort.

Hemostatic: Stops bleeding. Cayenne, mullein, goldenseal, yellow dock.

Hepatoprotective: Supports normal liver function. Burdock, dandelion, turmeric.

Hypotensive: Lowers blood pressure. Garlic, ginger, hawthorne, motherwort.

Immunomodulator: Assists the body's defense system, by strengthening the immune system. Astragalus, echinacea, garlic, St. John's wort.

Laxative: Promotes bowel movements. Dandelion, yellow dock.

Lymphagogue: Helps lymph system to cleanse and strengthen. Burdock, calendula, mullein, red clover.

Nervine: Calms the nerves. Chamomile, motherwort, valerian.

Nutritive: Nourishes and strengthens the entire system. Burdock, dandelion, nettle, plantain.

Sedative: Strong relaxing support to the nervous system. Valerian, chamomile, catnip, skullcap.

Stimulant: Increases energy. Echinacea, ginseng, dandelion, elecampane, sage.

Stomachic: See Bitter and Tonic.

Tonic: General promotion of functions of the entire body, or specific systems. Boosts energy on a deep level. Nettle, dandelion, burdock, ginseng, skullcap.

Vulnerary: Encourages the healing of wounds and irritated tissues. Aloe, comfrey, calendula.

APPENDIX 2

Additional Herbal Remedies

Here, we are including useful herbs and remedies for overall immune support, specifically to treat diseases of the gut. Ninety percent of our immune system lies in our gut, and diseases of this origin are very common now, and on the rise.

Herbal medicines for inflammatory bowel disease (IBD) combine anti-inflammatory herbs, demulcents, astringents, immune-enhancing herbs, and adaptogens. See *Living with Crohn's & Colitis* by Jessica Black and Dede Cummings for more information on herbal remedies and digestive wellness.

Anti-inflammatory herbs

Garlic is also a useful supplement especially if there is concern that there is yeast, bacterial, or parasitic overgrowth. Garlic is anti-inflammatory, blood thinning, anti-microbial, and anti-cancer. Garlic supplements need to be taken with the odor to get the best effect. Don't bother buying an odor-less garlic supplement, because you lose half of what makes garlic so powerful. If your stomach, family members, and co-workers can handle it, the best way to take garlic is to eat garlic cloves. One way to do this is by making a small drink.

Garlic Drink Recipe

1 clove garlic, minced small
½ glass filtered water
pure maple syrup, to taste
juice of half a lemon

Mix together and drink one of these drinks two times daily.

Try just eating garlic, as it is being studied more and more for its health effects and its reduction in colorectal cancer risk in inflammatory bowel disease sufferers. If you want to take garlic in capsule form, the proper dosage should be at least 900 mg daily. Some supplements can be found having high allicin content, which is the main constituent in garlic. These high allicin supplements are different than taking garlic supplements, therefore the mg dosage daily is much smaller.

Ginger can also be used alone especially for gastrointestinal irritation and inflammation. Ginger tea is helpful in settling the stomach and can also be helpful to alleviate nausea. Drink 3 cups of this tea daily.

Turmeric, or curcumin, can be used as a spice in foods or can be taken in therapeutic doses either through tincture form or capsule form. Curcumin has significant anti-inflammatory properties and very high antioxidant capability making it a superb nutrient to use in any gastrointestinal condition, inflammation-related condition, and to use preventatively to ward off cancer and chronic illness.

One of the most effective forms of curcumin is to take it in a tincture with ginger. Dr. Black's clinic uses a tincture called the "anti-inflammatory tincture," which is used for anything from inflammatory bowel disease to arthritis to acute injuries to chronic idiopathic inflammatory diseases. This tincture gets extremely positive results in almost all patients who begin taking it regularly. The proportion should be about 50/50 curcumin to ginger as they are both anti-inflammatory and the ginger helps with the absorption of curcumin. Because curcumin is poorly absorbed, it should be complexed either with ginger or bromelain for optimal absorption and optimal effects.

In people who have ulcerative colitis, previous studies have shown that curcumin supplements, when compared with a placebo, reduced the number of relapses by about 50 percent. A recent article in *Current Pharmaceutical Design* also notes that in the treatment of inflammatory bowel disease, curcumin "and its unrivalled safety profile suggest that it has bright prospects."

Turmeric complexed with ginger in liquid tincture form should be used as follows: 2 dropperfuls 3–4 times per day. Too much curcumin can cause stomach upset so don't use much more than this listed dosage. In capsule form, curcumin complexed with either ginger or bromelain can be taken at 500 mg of the curcumin 2–3 times daily. If you can't find a capsule of curcumin and ginger or curcumin and bromelain, you can always buy curcumin and ginger capsules separately and take them together to help with curcumin absorption and reduce gastrointestinal irritation.

Yucca is a plant native to Mexico and Southwestern United States. Yucca has been known in folk medicine as a treatment for arthritis and inflammatory ailments. Native American tribes and native peoples of Mexico have proclaimed many uses of yucca that have dated back hundreds of years. Yucca is comprised of many phytochemicals that make it special to use for many conditions. Some of the important phytochemicals are phenolic compounds such as resveratrol. Resveratrol is an important anti-inflammatory agent that helps reduce aging and helps to keep inflammation under control. The phenolic compounds in yucca also act as antioxidants or free radical scavengers that reduce damage and inflammation caused by free radicals, thereby reducing damage and aging of tissues, joints, organs, etc. Yucca is more often used in patients who have inflammatory bowel issues or gastrointestinal distress that coincides with

arthritis. Yucca is also high in saponins, which play a part in complexing with the cholesterol molecule in the body aiding in cholesterol lowering. This cholesterol lowering effect was demonstrated more than 45 years ago.

Yucca dosage should be two 500 mg tablets or capsules 2–3 times per day. It is always best to start at a lower dosage and increase if no result is seen. Yucca can also be found as a tea and will be mentioned in the tea section as well. The usual dosage for tea is 3–5 cups per day. Long-term high dosage use of yucca extract can result in interference with the absorption of vitamins A, D, E, and K.

Pau d'arco, or *Tabebuia impetiginosa*, contains at least 20 active compounds, including naphthaquinones, anthraquinones, alkaloids, quercetin, and other flavonoids. Flavonoids will help support and balance the immune response and inflammatory response and help to reduce the allergic response. Alkaloids are found in varying quantities in most plants and are the part of the plant that makes them have a bitter taste. Because large dosages of alkaloids can be toxic, this bitter taste, obviously more bitter in more toxic plants, can warn animals of the plant's toxic nature. This is one example why it is most helpful to use plants in their whole form as much as possible for treating illness. Using plants in their whole form will help ensure the amounts of toxic or irritating substances like alkaloids are surrounded by other balancing phytochemicals, ensuring subtle and effective medicinal effects. Alkaloids are a nitrogen-containing part of the plant that represent a very diverse group of significant compounds that include well-known drugs like the opiates, caffeine, nicotine, and quinine, the antimalarial drug.

Pau d'arco can be used as an immune system stimulant, and to decrease inflammation. It should only be used in inflammatory bowel disease patients if there is an underlying infection problem contributing to illness.

Pau d'arco can be found in capsules, tinctures, or as a tea. The tea is best, but it must be boiled slowly to gain all medicinal properties from the plant. The following dosages for capsules and tinctures should be discussed with your doctor prior to use:

- Capsules: 300–500 mg three times per day
- Tincture (1:5): 0.5–1 mL (about ⅛–¼ teaspoon) two or three times per day

To prepare pau d'arco tea, mix 3–6 tablespoons of the inner bark tea with one quart of cold distilled water into a teapot. This can be brought to a low boil for 20 minutes. Then strain and drink 3 cups daily.

Even low doses of pau d'arco can cause dizziness, nausea, vomiting, and diarrhea and can interfere with blood clotting. It may also cause skin sensitivity. The potential for drug-nutrient or nutrient-nutrient interactions should be considered when using pau d'arco. Don't use with other blood thinners unless supervised by a physician and if any side effects occur after its use, discontinue. Pau d'arco should be avoided in pregnancy and lactation. Pau d'arco should not be given to infants or children.

Cat's claw is a large woody vine indigenous to the Amazon rain forest of South America and is also known as *Uncaria tomentosa*. Its phytochemical makeup is important to its functions as well. The active compounds in cat's claw include alkaloids, triterpenes, phytosterols, and proanthocyanidins. Some of the phytochemicals in cat's claw appear to have anti-inflammatory, antioxidant, and anticancer effects. It is used in a wide variety of health issues including healing and treating digestive and intestinal disorders. The phytosterol component of the herb provides insight into how it can balance the immune response. Phytosterols are components of plants that are responsible in balancing the actions of the Th1 and Th2 systems and can play a significant role in reducing inflammation by balancing any overactive or underactive part of the immune response.

Bitters

Bitters are useful herbs that function to stimulate gastric function in addition to liver function and detoxification. They help to control blood sugar, and they aid in stress relief due to their stimulation of the parasympathetic nerves in the gastrointestinal tract. They are helpful in IBD patients because they stimulate mucosal immunity and function to create balance of inflammation within the GI tract and they may help to repair mucosal wall damage caused by inflammation.

Examples of bitters include licorice, peppermint, calendula, dandelion, artichoke leaf, blessed thistle, angelica, motherwort, wormwood, bitter orange peel, lemon peel, gentian root, mugwort, goldenseal, cascara sagrada, hops, chamomile, and yarrow.

An example of how to use bitters is before or after a meal. It can be in the form of a tincture or tea, but tincture is best considering it is easier to carry with you when you are out. A tincture of equal parts licorice, dandelion, and blessed thistle might be a good start. Use 2 dropperfuls with each meal. This may have to be taken in a little bit of water due to its strong and bitter taste.

Demulcents

A demulcent is an herb that functions in providing a soothing film over a mucus membrane. For example, honey is often

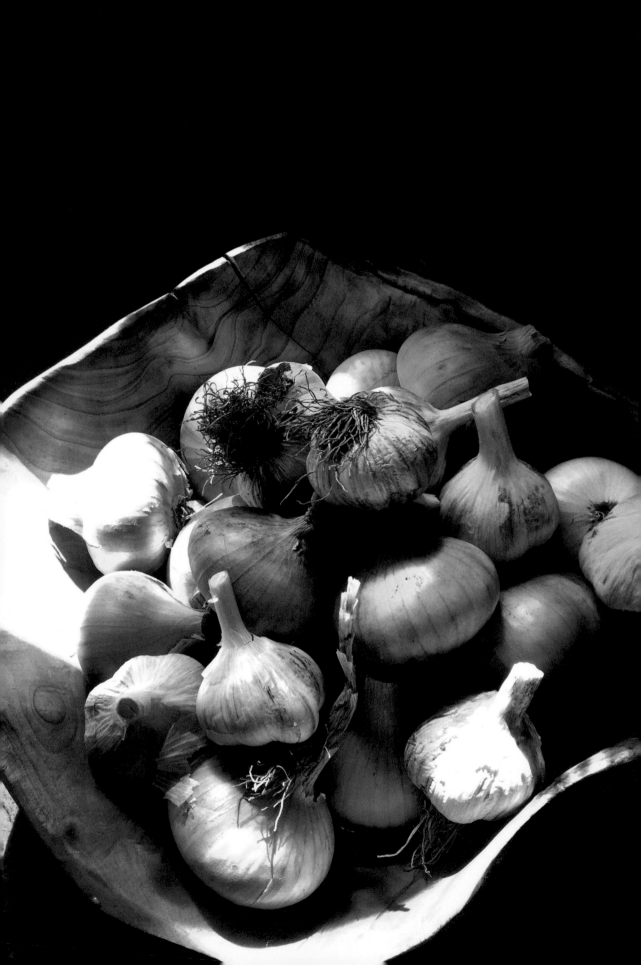

used as a demulcent for a sore throat, because it helps to coat the throat mucus membrane. Respiratory demulcent herbs can be extremely effective in treating coughs and soothing lung irritation.

The demulcent slippery elm can be very useful in calming, soothing, and coating the GI tract. Other soothing demulcents include comfrey, althaea, licorice, and matricaria, which can be used to help soothe gastrointestinal irritation.

Demulcents can be used as cold teas, tinctures, and capsules. It is best to use demulcents as warm or cold teas because they perform best that way.

Astringents

An astringent is used to help bring tissue together. It shrinks it together and can help with micro tears, micro bleeds, and excess mucus in the gastrointestinal tract. Some helpful astringents in IBD include agrimony, comfrey, geranium, yarrow, and lady's mantle. Most often, these are not used alone, but are used in combination with anti-inflammatory herbs, demulcents, and immune enhancing herbs.

Immune-enhancing herbs

One of the most important areas to support in autoimmune diseases is the immune system. We sometimes wrongly direct our treatments for autoimmune diseases by suppressing the immune response rather than balancing the immune response. Drugs targeted at T-lymphocyte regulation will be a fairly large area of research in the future. For now, we utilize herbs that help the body achieve better immune homeostasis such as astragalus, baical skullcap, chaparral, pau d'arco, albizia, reishi, shiitake, and other mushrooms.

One must be careful and skilled at using herbal medicine to treat the immune system in autoimmune diseases to ensure proper stimulation without overstimulating the wrong part of the immune system.

Adaptogens

Adaptogens refer to a class of herbs that help the body in its adaptation to its environment. Most of the time, adaptogens help to support the adrenal gland, which sits on top of the kidney and functions in our stress response. The adrenal glands help to control immune function, blood pressure, emotions, blood sugar, and importantly, control the output of our cortisol, which helps us feel energy for the day and modulates our immune response. Adaptogens are very useful in the beginning of illness to bring energy up, help individuals cope with stress, and to improve sense of well-being and sense of worth. This increased self-awareness and self-love helps patients focus on their treatment plans and increases compliance with new lifestyle and diet changes.

Examples of adaptogens are Siberian ginseng, withania, licorice, astragalus, rehmania, codonopsis, maca, rhodiola, schisandra, cordyceps, reishi mushroom, and noni. Use adaptogens in tincture form. Pick 2–4 herbs to add to a tincture in equal parts and dosing it at 2 dropperfuls 3 times per day. The last dose of the day should not be before bed, as adaptogens can often keep individuals from sleeping well.

Example Adaptogen Tincture for IBD

1 part Siberian ginseng
1 part maca
1 part rehmania
1 part codonopsis due to its effect on the gastrointestinal tract

If you can't find an herbalist or doctor who can make this tincture, then you can purchase four 1-ounce tinctures and mix them together into a 4-ounce dark container. Then you can pour 1 ounce back into one of the bottles, label it appropriately and this can be your dispensing bottle. If you can't find one of these herbs, then replace it with another of the adaptogens listed or omit it entirely. Before making an adaptogen formula read about the specifics of each adaptogen and determine which 3–4 adaptogens are most appropriate for you.

Teas for healing

IBD Tea for Mood, Nervine, and Calming

1 part St. John's wort (St. John's wort should not be used by people currently taking antidepressant medication)
1 part lemon balm
1 part passion flower

Steep 1 tablespoon per 10 ounces of water. Bring appropriate amount of water to boil, remove from heat, add dry herb, cover, and allow to steep for 15 minutes. Strain through a fine tea strainer, cheesecloth, or clean nylon/T-shirt. Drink 3 cups daily. You can make up to 90 ounces at once and sweeten with honey if desired. If you are making bigger batches, it is perfectly okay to store in the refrigerator and drink chilled.

IBD Tea for Detoxification and Soothing

1 part licorice root
1 part marshmallow root
1 part burdock root
1 part dandelion root
1 part yellow dock root

Yellow dock should not be used by people taking drugs that decrease blood calcium, such as diuretics, Dilantin, Miacalcin, or Mithracin. It also should not be used by people with kidney disease, liver disease, or an electrolyte abnormality.

Because these herbs are roots, the tea needs to be boiled to release the maximum medicinal qualities of the herbs. Add 1 tablespoon of the root mixture to 10 ounces of water. Bring water with herbs to a boil and boil for 10 minutes, remove from heat, cover, and allow to sit for 15 minutes. Strain and drink 3 cups daily. You can make up to 90 ounces at once and sweeten with honey if desired. If you are making bigger batches it is perfectly okay to store in the refrigerator and drink chilled.

IBD Tea for Inflammation and Immunity

1 part pau d'arco
1 part cat's claw
1 part ginger root—grated fine
1 part chaparral

Steep 1 tablespoon of the mixture per 14 ounces of water. Bring appropriate amount of water to boil, remove from heat, add dry herb, cover, and allow to steep for 15 minutes. Strain through a fine tea strainer, cheesecloth, or clean nylon/T-shirt. Drink 3 cups daily. You can make up to 90 ounces at once and sweeten with honey if desired. If you are making bigger batches, it is perfectly okay to store in the refrigerator and drink chilled.

IBD Soothing GI Tea

1 part dried peppermint leaves (use with care if you have heartburn or acid reflux)
1 part dried chamomile flowers

Steep 1 tablespoon per 10 ounces of water. Bring appropriate amount of water to boil, remove from heat, add dry herb, cover, and allow to steep for 15 minutes. Strain through fine tea strainer, cheesecloth, or clean nylon/T-shirt. Drink 3 cups

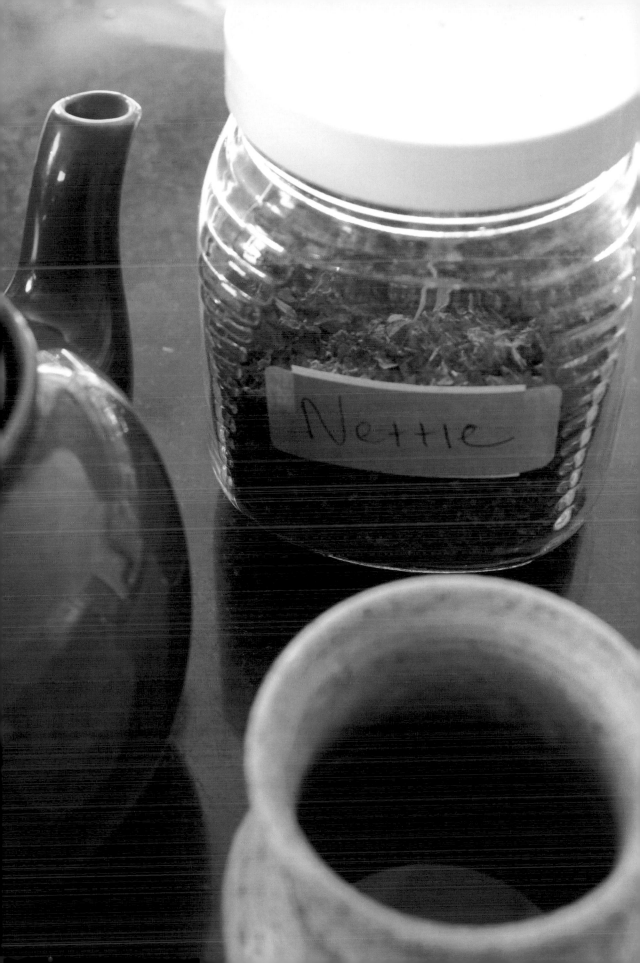

daily. You can make up to 90 ounces at once and sweeten with honey if desired. If you are making bigger batches it is perfectly okay to store in the refrigerator and drink chilled.

Chamomile

Steep 1 tablespoon per 10 ounces of water. Bring appropriate amount of water to boil, remove from heat, add dry herb, cover, and allow to steep for 15 minutes. Strain through a fine tea strainer, cheesecloth, or clean nylon/T-shirt. Drink 3 cups daily. You can make up to 90 ounces at once and sweeten with honey if desired. If you are making bigger batches, it is perfectly okay to store in the refrigerator and drink chilled.

IBD Gas Relief Tea

1 part fennel seeds—grind in coffee grinder slightly to help break apart the seed
1 part fenugreek seeds—grind in coffee grinder slightly to help break apart the seed
1 part althaea (marshmallow) root
1 part slippery elm bark—grind or break apart

Because these herbs are roots, seeds, and barks, the tea needs to be boiled to release the maximum medicinal qualities of the herbs. Add 1 tablespoon of the mixture to 10 ounces of water. Bring water with herbs to a boil and boil for 5–10 minutes, remove from heat, cover, and allow to sit for 15 minutes. Strain and drink 3 cups daily. You can make up to 90 ounces at once and sweeten with honey if desired. If you are making bigger batches, it is perfectly okay to store in the refrigerator and drink chilled.

Nutritional powders

Beneficial nutritional powders include spirulina, kelp, protein powders, brewer's yeast, ground nuts and seeds, acai powder, green tea powder, greens powder, ground milk thistle seeds, and ground nettle powder. As with everything, more is not always better. Moderation is the key to health; therefore do not begin including each of these powders in addition to many or all of the supplements listed.

Spirulina is a variety of seaweed that contains trace elements and minerals, essential fatty acids, increases absorption of iron and stimulates the immune system, cleanses and detoxifies, gently removes heavy metals, has enzymatic activity, is a vegetarian source of B-12, and contains a significant amount of beta-carotene.

Take one rounded tablespoon 2–3 times per day, this comes to around 30 grams daily. It is often suggested that you can take up to 100 grams daily. You can add this to water or a smoothie or juice and it doesn't change the taste significantly, but it certainly affects the color. My favorite way to consume spirulina is by drinking what we term in our home, "green lemonade."

Green Lemonade Recipe

1 cup filtered water
1 heaping tablespoon spirulina powder
½ teaspoon juice from a lemon
½ teaspoon pure maple syrup or honey

Stevia can be substituted for the syrup in this case.

Blend all the ingredients together in the blender until mixed. Enjoy 3 times per day (you can multiply the recipe by 3 to make 1 day's worth). Make fresh every day.

Kelp is another variety of seaweed and the powder can be beneficial to the gastrointestinal system due to its potential to regulate the thyroid, which is the organ that sets the pace of enzyme function in the body. The thyroid is our battery. How well it is functioning determines how optimally our enzymes can function. Remember that enzymes are important in the gastrointestinal tract for digesting foods and absorbing nutrients in addition to facilitating many metabolic reactions occurring within the gastrointestinal system, immune system, and the rest of the body. There are many health claims regarding the regular use of kelp including alleviating arthritis pain, increasing energy levels, stimulating immunity, improving glandular function, appetite control, and weight loss most likely due to optimizing metabolism. Kelp has been used to treat thyroid deficiency due to its rich iodine content. Kelp can help with poor digestion, flatulence, constipation, and helps to support mucus membrane health, which might give proof to its positive effect in inflammatory bowel disease patients. Kelp does have a distinct taste that is slightly salty. It can be used over food once daily.

Kelp powder: ½–1 teaspoon daily

Do not use if you have hyperthyroidism. Individuals who have hypothyroidism or borderline hypothyroidism may benefit most from daily use of kelp powder. The use of kelp may interfere with thyroid medication dosage requirements, therefore addition of daily kelp should be discussed with your physician and repeat thyroid tests should be performed six weeks after initiating kelp treatment.

Protein powders make a great addition for patients who need extra nutrition or need help balancing blood sugar. A protein shake can be added as a midmorning snack in between breakfast and lunch and can help to maintain stable blood sugars, stable moods, increased energy, and increased caloric intake for nutrient-deficient patients.

Brewer's yeast can be used to sprinkle over popcorn and most savory dishes. Brewer's yeast is made from Saccharomyces cerevisiae. Brewer's yeast is high in B vitamins, chromium, and many minerals. Due to its high chromium content, it may be helpful in reducing and balancing blood glucose levels and has also shown benefits in improving poor lipid profiles such as high cholesterol. Adults can use 1–2 tablespoons daily, but you might prefer to use brewer's yeast for a nutritive additive to some of your foods, rather than something that is consumed every day. There are much better supplements specific to lowering glucose or cholesterol.

Ground nuts and seeds can be added to many foods. You can use ground nuts and seeds for anything from raw dessert crusts, to pancakes, to crispy snack balls, to toppings for savory dishes. They add quality protein and fat to many recipes and are easily accessible at your local grocery store. Make sure to buy fresh nuts and seeds and organic if possible. Many nuts and seeds are also high in mineral content and will offer good sources of calcium and magnesium and many other important minerals.

Ground milk thistle seeds and ground nettle powder can be fun and beneficial additives to your foods. These powders can be mixed with salt to make a healthy seasoning for the table. Milk thistle helps to support liver function and nettle helps to support kidney function.

Good for Your Soul Salt

1 part ground milk thistle seeds
1 part ground nettle powder
1 part sea salt

Mix together and store in a salt shaker. Enjoy generously over food. This seasoning can be changed to fit your needs. For example, you can add kelp powder, sesame seeds, acai powder, and others to suit your needs and tastes.

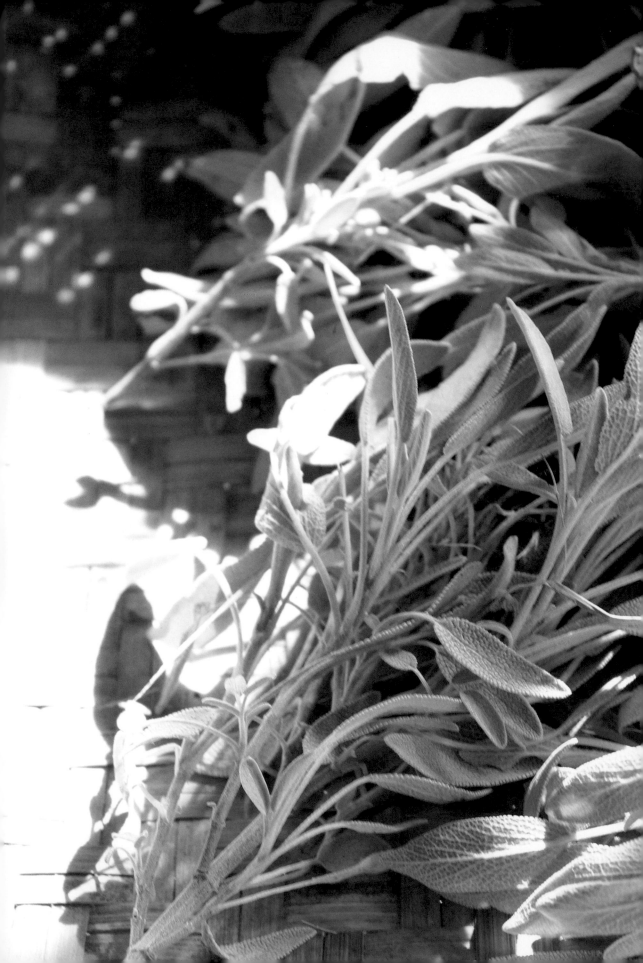

APPENDIX 3

Freezing Fresh Herbs

Freezing is an excellent way to preserve tender herbs, such as dill, basil, chives, parsley, and tarragon. It is very easy to freeze herbs, and it takes much less time than drying.

While it is possible to store herbs right out of the garden in the freezer, the quality in terms of taste and color will not be quite like fresh herbs; slightly bitter flavors and drab grayish-green colors are common. You can improve fresh herbs by blanching them before you freeze them. They still will not taste and look quite like fresh herbs, but they will come very close. It is best to use them while they're still frozen, but you can thaw frozen herbs in the refrigerator. When you thaw them in this way, they will keep for approximately one week.

To freeze fresh herbs:

- Rinse freshly picked herbs.
- Blanch for a few seconds using the following method:
  ° Bring 2–4 cups of water to a boil in any type of pot.
  ° Hold the herbs by their stems with tongs.
  ° Dip them in the boiling water briefly and swish them around a bit.
  ° When their color brightens, remove them from the water.
- Cool by using one of these methods:
  ° Hold them under running water and then blot them dry with a cloth or paper towels.
  ° Place them on towels after taking them from the boiling water to let them air cool.
- Remove stems, chop if desired or leave them with whole leaves that you can chop later.
- Freeze in one of these ways:
  ° Place in small plastic freezer bags in amounts that you are likely to use at one time.
  ° Place in ice cube trays and cover with water; repackage into freezer bags when frozen. (Note: if you use boiling water to cover your herbs, the hot cover not only protects the herbs from exposure to air, it also blanches them at the same time.)

To make it easier to separate your herbs when you want to use them later, lay the dried herbs out in a single layer on wax paper. Roll or fold the paper so that there is a layer of paper separating each layer of herb. Then, pack them, paper and all, in freezer bags or wrap in freezer-rated plastic wrap. To use, break off as much as you need, and chop them if you didn't do this earlier.

(From: www.four-h.purdue.edu/foods/Freezing%20fresh%20herbs.htm)

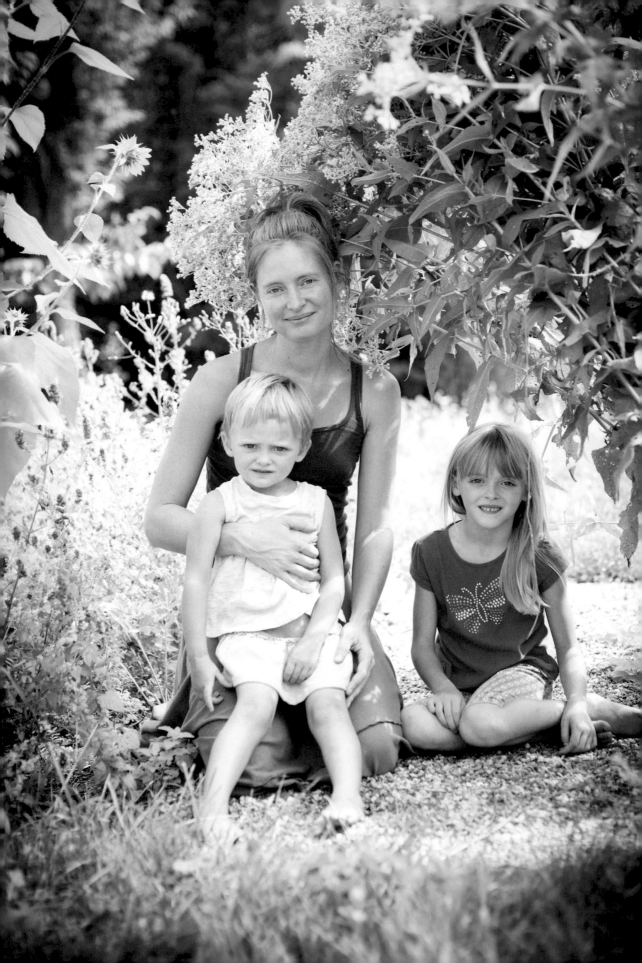

APPENDIX 4

Dosages

General adult dosages for long-term chronic problems such as insomnia, arthritis, pain, and allergies:

Infusion: 3–4 cups daily for 3–6 weeks.
Decoction: 1–2 cups daily for 3–6 weeks.
Syrup: 1–2 teaspoons 2 times daily.
Tincture: 2–3 dropperfuls 2–3 times daily for 3–6 weeks.
Capsule or pill ball: 2 pill balls 3 times a day for a month or two.

General adult dosages for acute, sudden illnesses such as flu, toothaches, headaches/migraine, burns, bleeding, and stomachache:

Infusion: ½ a cup at a time throughout the day—up to 4 cups total, until symptoms subside.
Decoction: ¼ cup at a time throughout the day—up to 2 cups total, until symptoms subside.
Syrup: 1 teaspoon every hour until symptoms subside.
Tincture: 1–2 dropperfuls every hour until symptoms subside.
Capsule or pill ball: 1 every hour until symptoms subside.

General dosages for children—based on the age:

2–4 years old—⅛ of an adult dose
4–6 years old— ¼ of an adult dose
6–8 years old—½ of an adult dose
8–10 years old—¾ of an adult dose
10 and up—adult dose most often will be good, but you may want to modify it taking into consideration your child's weight and their reaction to the dose.

These suggested dosages are to be used as a general guide, with modications made as needed. For acute symptoms, lower the dose by half, and administer every hour as needed.

Alyssa with her two daughters,
Patience and Sage

APPENDIX 5

Collecting Herbs in the Wild

For•age
verb
(of a person or animal) search widely for food or provisions

"Gulls are equipped by nature to **forage** for food."

Foraging for wild herbs is satisfying and worthwhile, but it's important to learn which plants are edible before you start ingesting anything . . . and to have fun in the process.

Learning how to forage for wild herbs and plants is also a way to educate your children about wild things in nature and conservation because many plants, such as echinacea, are endangered, so if we learn about foraging, we can really cover our bases while respecting the planet we live on.

Wild herbs and roots, like dandelion greens, are easy to identify and a good place to start. The dandelion plant is great to use as a diuretic and has lots of vitamins and nutrients.

Our ancestors foraged for herbs and cultivated herbs as well. In the area of northern New England where the authors live, the Algonquin Native Americans used herbs for all their medicinal needs, and they collected sap from trees and made their own maple syrup. The Algonquin Indians called it *sinzibukwud*, meaning "drawn from wood."

Whether you are foraging for herbs for medicinal uses or food to eat in the wild, one main advantage to doing this is learning a bit about what it was like to live life without all the modern luxuries and packaging, while getting some fresh air and appreciating the beauty found in nature.

When venturing out to collect herbs in wild places (wild crafting), we need to be mindful of the environment, the population, and health of the plant we are seeking to harvest; the time of year; the weather; tools we may need; and if it will be a long day, our own supplies of food and first aid! Wild crafting can be anything from picking a plantain leaf right from your front lawn to tromping through the forest all day to find cohosh to picking St. John's wort flowers from the farm field across the road. It can be a daily practice or a once-in-a-while adventure. Wild crafting can be so much fun, can bring a sense of oneness with nature, create awareness of your surroundings, and be just generally a wonderful way to bring the plants into your life.

When one is foraging, it's really important to note that some things are not edible, so it's good to go with someone who has some experience. It is also a good idea to take two baskets with you—one for herbs you know for sure, the other for new species that you want to get checked out from an expert before ingesting. It is helpful to learn the difference between certain herbs and edible plants—fragrance, leaves, flowers, etc., are all identifiers—and pick a small sample to start with and keep a notebook and photo portfolio.

There are some great websites to help with identifying as well.

Another advantage about foraging for herbs is that it is free! Things like bloodroot, coltsfoot, and mugwort also grow wild and abundantly along roadsides—but don't pick the herbs that are in heavy car traffic areas. Another cause for concern is for the herbs themselves: Never pick more than a small portion to ensure the plant has plenty of room to grow and propagate. The bonus about foraging for wild herbs is that they are usually abundant and readily available. Learn about what herbs or plants are endangered, and find out what is abundant and grows all around you as a way to get started. *A Field Guide to Edible Wild Plants* by Lee Allen Peterson is one of my favorite guides to foraging. It covers Eastern- and Central US and is well organized.

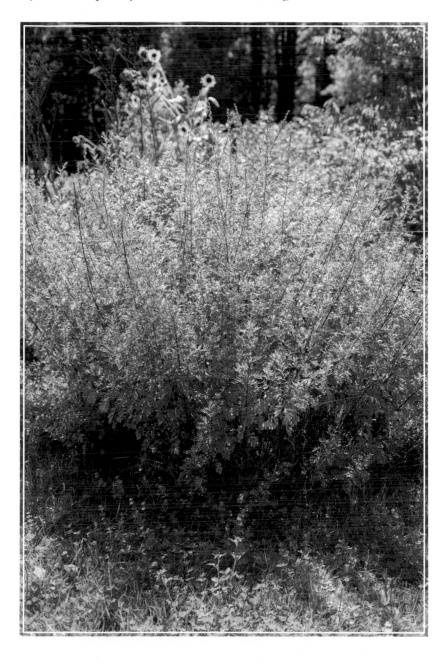

APPENDIX 6

Cooking with Herbs

The kitchen is bustling with activity. There are onions simmering in a cast-iron pan on the gas stove; a friend, or spouse, or child is chopping celery, peppers, and carrots on the counter; there is music playing on the stereo and lots of laughter and talking. Whether you are in a Vermont kitchen on a dirt road with not even the neighbors' lights for company, or in an urban kitchen somewhere far away, the act of cooking and sharing food remains the same.

This book espouses the practice of growing our own herbs, learning about them, and using them to actually heal our bodies. Whether growing a few herbs in your kitchen to augment your spice cabinet, add to the bath, or dry for healing tea, the practice and focus of your own path to herbal remedies is really what works for you. It is quite easy to start a garden at home or in a sunny window in your kitchen.

Why bother growing herbs in the first place? Medicinal herbs are the future and the past all in one; they hold the key to future cures, and have been around for centuries. When herbs are introduced into a family's lifestyle through cooking, the benefits are myriad in terms of health.

As we said in our introduction, bringing the herbs inside after harvesting fills your house with their aroma and beauty. Cooking with herbs is a whole new way to utilize their health benefits and bring exciting flavors into your meals!

Daily diet

In your daily life, try to eat the freshest, least-processed foods available, and the "locavore" movement is a way to participate on a community level. By "locavore" we mean food that is grown and produced within a 50-mile radius of where you live—food that is not shipped from so far away that it loses much of its nutritional value before it arrives.

By shifting to an herb-friendly diet, the body will not only be receiving rich nutrients, but will also become more balanced as there are many herbs that actually calm the digestive tract and soothe the process of elimination of the body's waste products.

Increasing the intake of the right fruits, vegetables, grains, and meats while staying away from sugary and over-processed foods can lead to better well-being. Some of the instructions for cooking with herbs in this section will also hopefully keep your health on track for years to come, and bring much joy into your life.

How to use fresh herbs in cooking

Remember that eating should be a pleasant experience, and eating well doesn't have to be a daunting task. Fresh herbs from your garden or farmer's market, fruits and vegetables, lean, locally-raised organic meats (or wild-caught and sustainably harvested fish), when eaten plain or in a delicious recipe, can brighten your day.

The more distance the food travels from farm to table, the greater the cost. Join a food co-op. Co-ops purchase food in bulk and often carry organic items. If there isn't one in your town, consider starting one with family and friends. Also, look for a local CSA (Community Supported Agriculture) farm stand in your area, where you can shop for local and organic vegetables, free-range chicken eggs, and broiler chickens on a weekly basis. Riding your bike or walking to the farm share is a great way to do the weekly pickups!

Organic food, grown in your garden or local farm

Everyone knows that eating foods that are free of pesticides, chemicals, antibiotics, colorings, or hormones is better for you. If you are not financially strained, make an effort to shop organic at your local farmers' market, growers, and stores. If budget is an issue, do not stress about it. Sometimes we have to make practical decisions and, understandably, eating organic may not always be the top priority. Also, keep in mind that due to very strict regulations, many farmers and growers are not able to obtain the organic label but are still producing foods that are free of pesticides, chemicals, antibiotics, and hormones, and are of excellent quality. All you need to do is find those products in your local stores and read their labels carefully.

Most of our readers can cook—we know that! However, this section will talk a bit more about the healing power of cooking with herbs and how to use them. Whether you use just a dash of a dried herb, or a beautiful fresh leaf from a peppermint plant, herbs can add zest and color to a dish.

1. **Basil** is one of the best herbs for culinary use. It is an herb that is relatively easy to grow and can be purchased at farmer's markets and grocery stores easily in bulk, too. In many kitchens, the end of the summer brings on the making of pesto, or *pistou* in French. This paste-like sauce is great over grilled veggies or tossed over fresh pasta, especially when paired with fresh-picked tomatoes. Basil has many healing properties as well—it's an immune booster and you can boil the leaves in water and mix in a little honey to soothe a sore throat. In the Ayurvedic healing modality, basil is an important herb. Chopping or picking fresh basil unleashes its scent, and the kitchen—and your nose—is filled with it.

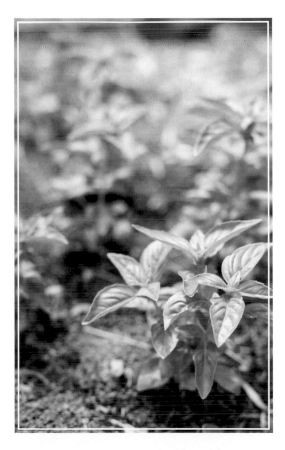

2. **Mint** is a wonderful addition to a cool glass of iced tea, used as a garnish for desserts, or chopped and used in cooking (fresh local lamb burgers and Raita, which is yogurt mixed with chopped cucumber and flavored with fresh chopped mint, are favorites).

3. **Rosemary** is a wonderful plant to have fresh, right in your kitchen. It is sometimes called "Dew of Sea" and comes from the Mediterranean. You can pick the fresh sprigs and chop them up finely on a cutting board to unleash the flavors—great to use in stews and with meat dishes!

4. **Oregano** and **thyme** grow wild, but you can also cultivate these wonderful herbs in your garden and sprinkle on salads, for example, or use in salad dressings and for flavoring dishes, like Italian-style tomato sauce, or soups. Oregano is a useful herb to steep and inhale when you have a cold!

5. **Cilantro** is an herb that some people adore while others run away from! It is great to have in the garden, and easy to grow. A wonderful addition to tacos, or dishes from the Mid-East, to add flavor and a sense of the exotic. You can add this beneficial herb to smoothies, too, to take advantage of its anti-inflammatory powers.

6. **Parsley** is one of our favorite herbs for cooking! Again, it's easy to grow and when used fresh it makes dishes come alive. Dede always chops fresh parsley and basil up to add to her lasagna that she makes with fresh spinach and local, fresh mozzarella. Another great plant to have growing in your kitchen year round! It is great to use as a garnish.

7. **Chives**. Well, nothing is better than a fresh dug potato, baked with butter and chopped chives. That's it. This herb is also easy to grow and has lots of Vitamin C. It is a great breath freshener!

8. **Dill** has the most delicate leaves and gets very tall in the garden, and sometimes unruly. But you can't beat the flavor! Dill is amazing to add to salad dressings, or our favorite, potato salads. Let's not forget dill pickles!

9. **Sage** is another Mediterranean herb that adds a smoky or musty flavor to dishes. It is great for digestion, and in Chinese medicine it is said to boost brainpower! At Dede's house, her son likes to use it in meat dishes to add flavor.

10. **Tarragon** is not something we grow around here, but for an exotic treat you can buy it and use it in Asian dishes and for a garnish. It is best thrown into a dish after the cooking is complete, or used as a garnish.

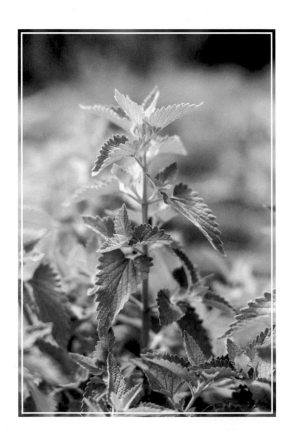

Recipes

Simple Pesto Soup
Serves 4–6

1 tablespoon butter
1 medium onion, diced
1 leek, diced
2 large tomatoes, peeled, seeded, and crushed
4 cups vegetable stock, *or* water
½ pound fresh green beans, chopped into bite-sized pieces
3 potatoes, chopped into bite-sized pieces
salt and pepper
¼ pound spaghetti
2 cloves garlic
several basil leaves
2 tablespoons olive oil
4 tablespoons grated Parmesan cheese

In a heavy medium-sized pot over medium-low heat, melt butter and slowly cook onion and leek. Add tomatoes. Add vegetable stock (or water) to pot and bring to a boil. Add green beans and potatoes. Season with salt and pepper. When veggies are almost cooked (about 15 minutes), add a handful of spaghetti (about ¼ pound), broken in half. Reduce heat and finish cooking very slowly.

Meanwhile, with a mortar and pestle, pound garlic with several basil leaves. While you're pounding, add olive oil, then 2–3 tablespoons of the soup broth. Serve soup, dividing pesto and grated Parmesan cheese between portions.

Chicken Stew
Serves 8–10

2 whole chickens, cut into pieces
2 cups red or white wine
3 tablespoons butter
3 tablespoons extra virgin olive oil
about 2 cups unbleached flour
2 teaspoons salt
2 teaspoons pepper
3 tablespoons butter
4 cups chicken stock
several sprigs fresh thyme, tied together
2–3 small pieces lemon peel
1 teaspoon dried green peppercorns, crushed
10–15 small red potatoes
1 pound fresh mushrooms
2 pounds medium boiling onions
4 tablespoons butter
4 tablespoons extra virgin olive oil
2 tablespoons parsley, finely chopped

Mix chicken pieces with wine and marinate in the refrigerator for 4 to 12 hours. Dry pieces well with paper towels, reserving marinade. Make a mixture of flour, salt and pepper. Melt 3 tablespoons butter and 3 tablespoons olive oil in a large, flameproof casserole. Dredge chicken pieces in flour mixture and brown on both sides in butter and oil over medium heat, a few at a time, reserving on a plate. Pour out browning fat and melt 3 tablespoons butter in the casserole. Add about ¼ cup of the flour mixture and cook, stirring constantly, for several minutes or until flour becomes lightly browned. Add wine marinade and chicken stock to casserole, blending well using a wire whisk. Bring to a boil and skim. Add thyme, peppercorns, lemon peel and chicken pieces to the pot, cover and bake at 325 degrees for about 2 hours. One hour before serving, add potatoes to the casserole.

Meanwhile, wash the mushrooms, dry well and sauté them, whole or sliced, in 2 tablespoons each of butter and olive oil. Peel the onions and sauté them gently in the remaining 2 tablespoons butter and 2 tablespoons olive oil for about 20 minutes. Just before serving, add mushrooms and onions to the casserole and stir in chopped parsley.

—*from Sally Fallon's* Nourished Cooking *(New Trends Publishing, 2001)*

Coconut Chicken Soup
Serves 4

1 quart chicken stock
1½ cups whole coconut milk, or 7 ounces creamed coconut
¼ teaspoon dried chile flakes
1 teaspoon freshly grated ginger
juice of 1 lemon
sea salt, or fish sauce
several green onions, very finely chopped (optional garnish)
1 tablespoon finely chopped cilantro (optional garnish)

Bring the stock to a boil, skim any foam that rises to the top, add coconut milk or creamed coconut, lemon juice, chile flakes, and ginger. Simmer for about 15 minutes. Season to taste with salt or fish sauce. Ladle into soup bowls or mugs and garnish with green onions or cilantro.

—*from Sally Fallon's* Nourished Cooking
(New Trends Publishing, 2001)

Chicken Rice Soup
Serves 6

2 quarts chicken stock
1 cup brown rice, preferably soaked for 7 hours
1 cup finely diced chicken meat and/or chicken liver and heart (leftover from making stock)
1½ cups finely diced vegetables such as carrot, celery, red pepper or string beans
sea salt, or fish sauce
pepper

Bring stock and rice to a boil and skim off any foam that may rise to the top. Reduce heat and cook, covered, about 1 hour until rice is tender. Add the vegetables, diced meats, season to taste and cook until just tender, about 5 to 10 minutes. Children love this!

—*from Sally Fallon's* Nourished Cooking
(New Trends Publishing, 2001)

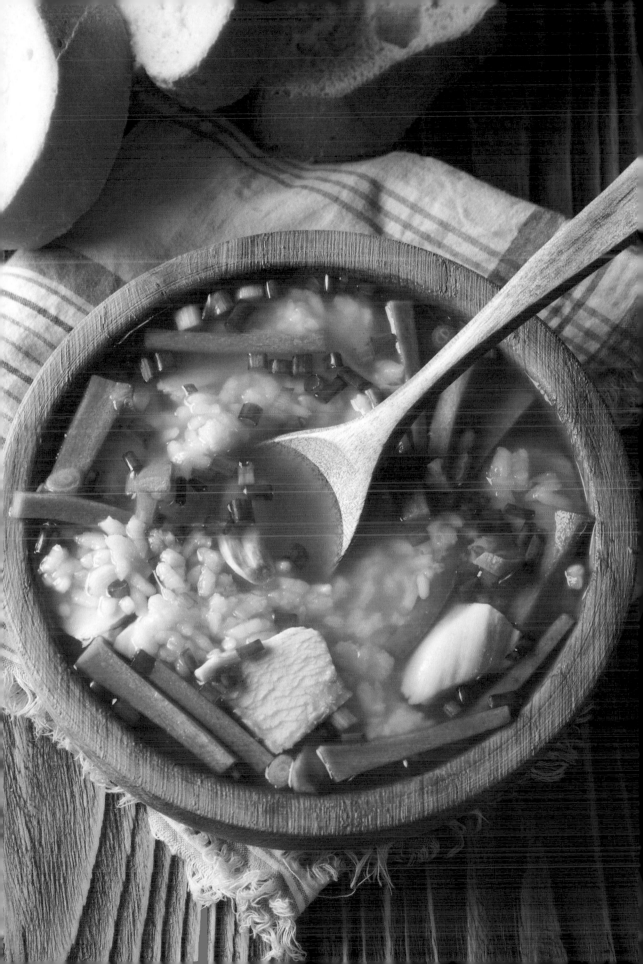

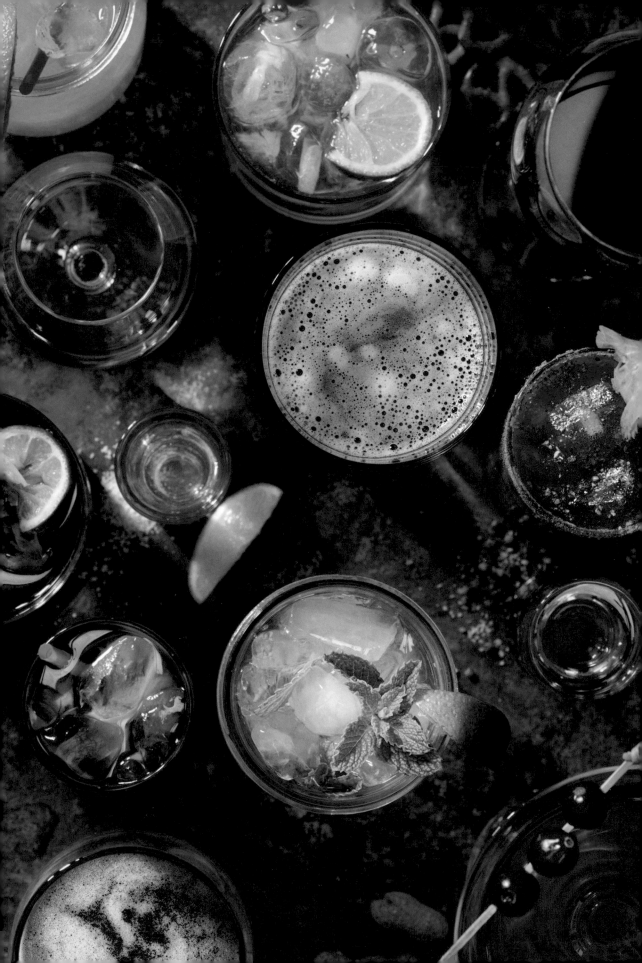

APPENDIX 7

Herbal Cocktails

Whether it's a cold winter night in snowy Vermont, or an urban backyard in the spring, or a beach picnic in the summertime, a cocktail with friends and family can be an enjoyable experience, with or without alcohol. So why not add healthy ingredients to boost your system and support your liver while you're at it?

Note: Adjust ingredients and alcohol amounts to one's liking.

Healing Spiced Rum and Soda

2 ounces cooled cinnamon-astragalus
   decoction
1 shot rum
2 ounces root beer
2 ounces seltzer

Gin-Gin and Lime

2 ounces cooled ginger decoction
1 shot gin
3 ounces seltzer
1 ounce lime juice

Purple Boost

1 ounce elderberry syrup
1 shot vodka
5–7 ounces seltzer

Cape Codder Stress Relief

1 tablespoon muddled tulsi and lavender
1 shot vodka
5–7 ounces cranberry juice

Dandelion White Russian

2 ounces cooled roasted dandelion root
   decoction
1 shot Kahlúa*
Desired amount of milk, cream, or dairy-
   free alternative of choice

*For the Kahlúa, you can either buy the brand or make your own:
   2½ cups strong, freshly brewed coffee
   2 cups maple syrup (can use honey
     if desired)
   2¼ cups good quality vodka
   1 vanilla bean, cut into thirds
  Make the coffee. Add maple syrup (or honey) and let cool. Add vodka and pour into glass jar with vanilla bean cuttings. Label and store jar in the fridge for 30 days, and it will be ready to drink.

Healing Toddy

1 ounce echinacea-ginger syrup
1 shot whiskey
1 ounce lemon juice
Desired amount of water
(enjoyed hot or cold)

APPENDIX 8

The Healing Power of Mushrooms

"Mushrooms are forest guardians. A forest ecosystem cannot be defined without its fungi because they govern the transition between life and death and the building of soils, all the while fueling numerous life cycles."

—Paul Stamets, *Mycelium Running;
How Mushrooms Can Help Save the World*

Mushrooms serve so many purposes and are incredibly healing on many levels. In nature, they cover most of the earth, even in places where we don't see the actual flowering or fruiting bodies of the plant, the mycelium—the network of fungi underneath the ground—is everywhere, and what it does is quite beneficial and intriguing. Mushrooms aerate the soil, bringing nutrients through it to plants or areas that are in need, literally! They communicate through the mycelium network—think of it like our nervous system—to deliver what is needed through the forest ecosystem, and even to other forests miles away.

Mushrooms breathe oxygen. Think about this. Plants breathe carbon dioxide. Mushrooms are more like animals than plants in a lot of ways, and it's interesting how much they go unnoticed, or undervalued. They are an intricate part of the health of this planet, and many cultures throughout history have known this, used them as food and medicine, and valued them highly.

Mushrooms are being used for eco-restoration and bioremediation on small and massive scales today. They are being used to clean up toxic waste, nuclear fallout, to rebuild depleted soils that are leading to catastrophic erosion, and to bring over-logged/compacted tracts of land areas back to life. The potential is growing, as more people become interested and aware of this use for mushrooms and learn how easy it is to make a difference in the environment with the use of them. They are relatively easy to cultivate and spread rapidly, thus getting to know the damage around them, only to speedily clean it up. Absolutely amazing.

If mushrooms can heal the planet on this level, it's no wonder they can heal our bodies as well. Various types of mushrooms are healing for various diseases and used for overall longevity and vibrant health. There are culinary varieties and varieties that are more medicinal. Many studies have been and are being done all over the world regarding the treatment of cancers with mushrooms. This is very exciting. The cell normalizing abilities of mushrooms is powerful, and if taken in the right dosages with the right professional guidance, can be extremely beneficial for patients of all types. The other beautiful thing about mushroom medicine is that it often can be taken alongside other drugs and herbs to further potentiate their effects.

For the purpose of this book, let's look more deeply into the healing properties and growing/wild crafting of mushrooms on a small home scale.

Mushrooms can be easily cultivated by getting the spores and inoculating them into the right medium (see Resources for specifics). They are all a little bit different—some like to grow in logs, some in woodchips in a patch on the ground, and some in manure and straw. Once there is a patch growing nearby, certain species—such as oyster mushrooms—can be transplanted throughout the garden, and will thrive, not minding the sun exposure. This brings much health to any garden, not only because you get to harvest the mushroom fruits themselves, but they bring nutrients to the soil, make space in compacted soil, and all of these functions actually help produce noticeably larger and healthier plants in and around the garden. Most of the time we are growing mushrooms in our gardens whether we know it or not! And when we do see them popping up here and there, especially after a rain storm or during a wet season, we can be comforted in knowing they are there to help, even if they are not a type we want to use for food or medicine. Speaking of which, it is very important to not harvest mushrooms that are not absolutely positively identifiable! There are poisonous species out there, so please do not take a chance.

A Few Edible and Medicinal Mushroom Profiles

Chanterelle
Cantharellus cibarius

Chanterelles are visually appealing and very tasty. They are fairly common, and easy to find from July through September, sometimes growing in massive abundance. They range from pale yellow to dark orange in color, and look like small trumpets.

They are best used fresh in cooking, and are most commonly used in preparation with meats, vegetables, rice, pasta, or potatoes. They can be made into a nice sauce by sautéing with onions and adding cream.

Oyster
Pleurotus ostreatus

Oyster mushrooms can be found in fall to early winter growing on dying trees or rotting logs. They are delicious and have medicinal properties as well. They have a strong anise-like aroma, but as they get older develop an unpleasant smell. They have a tan to gray-blue like color. For cooking, they are highly recommended for tempura. There have been studies that indicate oyster mushrooms may be useful in the treatment of prostate and other cancers.

Maitake
Grifola frondosa

Also known as Hen of the Woods—not to be confused with Chicken of the Woods, Laetiporus sulphureus. In addition to being a nice edible, Maitake is highly medicinal, used to boost the immune system, fight cancer (the Sloan Kettering Cancer Center is conducting ongoing studies and the American Cancer Society has positive things to say about this species), and stabilize blood pressure and blood sugar. They can be found from August to November, mostly on and at the base of dying oak trees, or in areas where there are oak trees. Delicious sautéed, fried, or boiled. They freeze and dry well for later use.

Yellow Morels
Morchella esculenta

Warning: Never eat a raw morel, or a false morel! Make sure to find a good resource with clear photos to positively identify the right one.

They are delicious sautéed, deep fried, or dried and reconstituted. They are nice prepared with fish as well, and make a good addition to a soup. Morels are most often found in old orchards that are no longer farmed and are full of unmanaged trees. Also found often among berry bushes, near wood chip piles and compost, along field edges, and near gardens. Can be found from the beginning of April through mid-June.

Puffballs
Calvatia gigantea

When harvesting, make sure the puffball is as large or larger than your fist. This ensures safety as it can be mistaken for amanita buttons (toxic) when small. Large, spherical, and whitish in color, they are often found fruiting one at a time, sometimes in groups. Can be found in late spring or fall among lawns, fields, field edges, and occasionally under hardwood trees. Puffballs are great sliced thinly and sautéed.

Reishi
Ganoderma tsugae

Very common in the northeast, these often grow on old hemlock trees or stumps. They are kidney-shaped and go from white to orange to golden brown at the base. Waxy and tough, reishi mushrooms are used in medicine, but not so much in cooking. Found from spring to fall.

Commonly made into a tincture or liquor (see resources). Useful in treating some cancers, especially breast cancer. May have negative interactions with some medications, so check with your doctor.

Turkey Tail
Trametes versicolor

Probably the most common wild mushroom, turkey tails grow on many types of rotting stumps, logs, and trees. They are highly medicinal and used in the treatment of colorectal cancer and leukemia, as an adjunct therapy. They look like turkeys tails, and are found throughout the whole growing season. They are tough and leathery. They can be dried, ground, and made into a decoction/tincture (see Resources).

Chaga
Inonotus obliquus

Chaga looks like a large blackish canker, most often found growing on birch trees. It can be found all year long, often growing for many years. It is highly medicinal, usually being made into a tea or tincture. Quite tasty, similar to coffee, it has been used as a tonic and a cancer treatment in Russia for thousands of years.

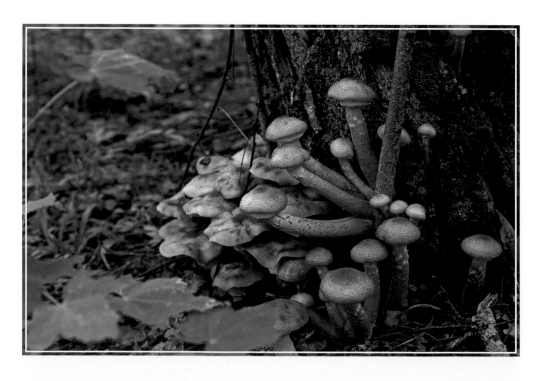

RESOURCES

Companies/Organizations

Alchemical Solutions
www.organicalcohol.com
700 Mistletoe Road, Suite 101, Ashland, OR
97520
   Organic 190-proof alcohol in bulk quantities for making tinctures. Grain, grape, cane,
and corn alcohols available.

American Herb Association
www.ahaherb.com
   Provides an herb calendar of events that
lists herbal, foraging, and aromatherapy
events throughout North America. A great
newsletter you can subscribe to with topics
such as herb gardening, Chinese medicine,
ayurveda, clinical herbalism, ethnobotany,
and wild crafting.

American Herbalists Guild
www.americanherbalistguild.com
   A nonprofit, educational organization to
represent the goals and voices of herbalists
specializing in the medicinal use of plants.
Promotes a high level of professionalism
and education in the study and practice of
therapeutic herbalism. This is a great organization to be a part of for our readers who
are thinking about—or already are—practic-
ing herbalism professionally.

Courtney Wilder
(212) 461-2577
Courtywilder@yahoo.com
   Diversified urban landscape gardener in
New York City.

FEDCO Seeds
www.fedcoseeds.com
PO Box 520, Waterville, ME 04903
   Seeds and grower's supplies, including
tools, books, pots, soil, compost, etc. They
have a really fun catalog and are a cooperative!

Fungi Perfecti
www.hostdefense.com
PO Box 7634, Olympia, WA 98507
877-504-6926
   Medicinal Mushroom Products formulated
by Paul Stamets.

High Meadows Farm
www.highmeadowsfarm.com
742 Westminster West Road, Putney, VT
05346
   Many high-quality organic potted herbs.

Horizon Herbs
www.horizonherbs.com
PO Box 69, Williams, OR 97544
(541) 846-6704
   Seeds, plants, roots, bulbs, tubers, seed
cleaning screens, tincture presses, dried bulk
herbs, herbal products,
and books.

Mountain Rose Herbs
www.mountainroseherbs.com
PO Box 50220, Eugene, OR 97405
(800) 879-3337
   Bulk organic herbs and spices, carrier
and essential oils, butters and waxes, herbal
encapsulaters, bottles, salts, teas, herbal
products, books, and more.

**Sage Mountain Retreat Center and
Botanical Sanctuary**
www.sagemountain.com
PO Box 420, East Barre, VT 05649
   Study courses, retreats, workshops, confer-
ences, and events, Herbal products. Home of
Rosemary Gladstar, world-renowned herbal-
ist extroadinaire.

Specialty Bottles
www.specialtybottle.com
   Bottles and jars—glass, plastic, and tin.
Discounts on bulk quantities.

Sungro Horticulture

www.sungro.com

770 Silver Street, Agawam, MA 01001

Suppliers of Metro Mix and Fafard soil mixes and other products for container gardening.

United Plant Savers

www.unitedplantsavers.org

An organization devoted to protecting medicinal plants in the United States and Canada and their native habitat while ensuring an abundant renewable supply of medicinal herbs for generations to come. You can become a member and recieve seeds to plant that are endangered or at risk, the oppurtunity to make your garden a certified Botanical Sanctuary, and other resources and information regarding sustainable plant medicine.

Zack Woods Herb Farm

www.zackwoodsherbs.com

278 Mead Road, Hyde Park, VT 05655

(802) 888-7278

Bulk herbs and herbal products, tours, workshops, classes. Owned and operated by Rosemary Gladstar's daughter Melanie and her husband Jeff.

Books

Breedlove, Greta, *The Herbal Home Spa: Naturally Refreshing Wraps, Rubs, Lotions, Masks, Oils, and Scrubs*, Storey Publishing, LLC, 9th edition (1998).

Cech, Richo, *Making Plant Medicine*, Horizon Herbs (2000).

Cummings, Dede (with Jessica Black, ND), *Living with Crohn's & Colitis: A Comprehensive Naturopathic Guide for Complete Digestive Wellness*, Hatherleigh Press (2010).

Gladstar, Rosemary, *Family Herbal: A Guide to Living Life with Energy, Health, and Vitality*, Storey Publishing, LLC (2001).

Gladstar, Rosemary, *Herbal Healing for Women*, Touchstone (1993).

Harrod Buhner, Stephen, *Herbal Antibiotics: Natural Alternatives for Treating Drug-Resistant Bacteria*, Storey Publishing, LLC, 2nd edition (2012).

Hobbs, Chris, *Medicinal Mushrooms: An Exploration of Tradition, Healing, and Culture*, Book Pub Co (2003).

Hoffman, David, *The New Holistic Herbal*, Element Books Ltd. (1991).

Kavasch, E. Barrie. *The Medicine Wheel Garden: Creating Sacred Space for Healing, Celebration, and Tranquility.* Bantam (2002).

Organic Gardening Magazine, The Rodale Encyclodedia of Organic Gardening, Rodale Books (1993).

Parvati, Jeannine, *Hygieia: A Woman's Herbal*, North Atlantic Books (2010).

Peterson, Lee Allen, *A Field Guide to Edible Wild Plants: Eastern and Central North America*, Houghton Mifflin Harcourt (1999).

Remen, Rachel Naomi, MD, *Kitchen Table Wisdom: Stories That Heal*, Riverhead Trade Books (1997).

Scott, Timothy Lee, *Invasive Plant Medicine: The Ecological Benefits and Healing Abilities of Invasives*, Healing Arts Press (2010).

Seymour, John, *The Self-Sufficient Gardener: A Complete Guide to Growing and Preserving All Your Own Food*, Doubleday (1979).

Spahr, David L., *Edible and Medicinal Mushrooms of New England and Eastern Canada*, North Atlantic Books (2009).

Stamets, Paul, *Growing Gourmet and Medicinal Mushrooms*, Ten Speed Press (2000).

Stamets, Paul, *Mycelium Running: How Mushrooms Can Help Save the World*, Ten Speed Press (2005).

Tierra, Michael, *The Way of Herbs*, Pocket Books, revised edition (1998).

Tilgner, Sharol, *Herbal Medicine from the Heart of the Earth*, Wise Acres LLC, 2nd edition (2009).

Tourles, Stephanie, *The Herbal Body Book: A Natural Approach to Healthier Hair, Skin, and Nails*, Storey Publishing, LLC (1994).

Weed, Susun S., *Healing Wise*, Ash Tree Publishing (2003).

Weed, Susun S., *Wise Woman Herbal for the Childbearing Year*, Ash Tree (1996).

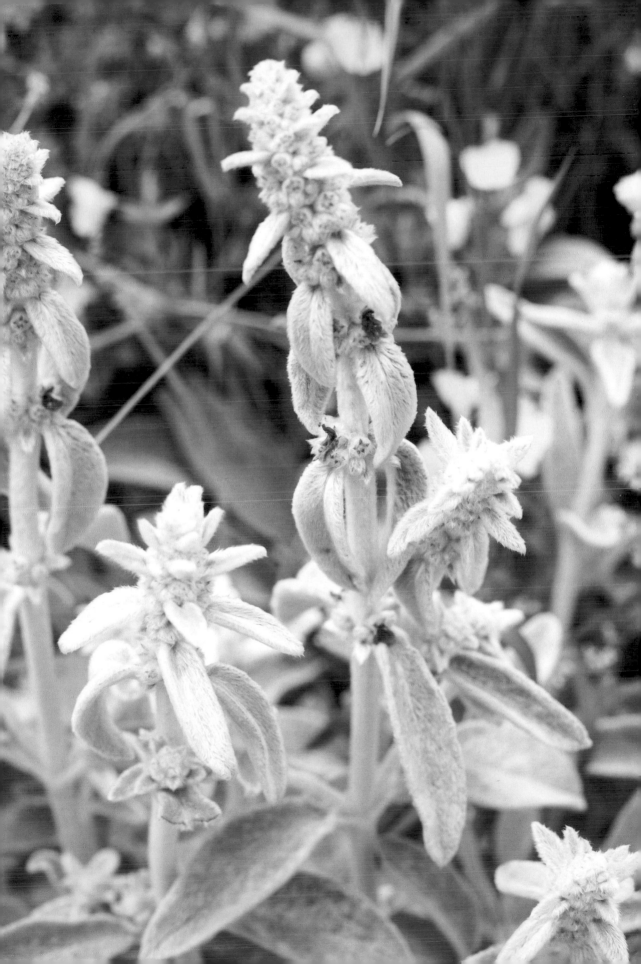

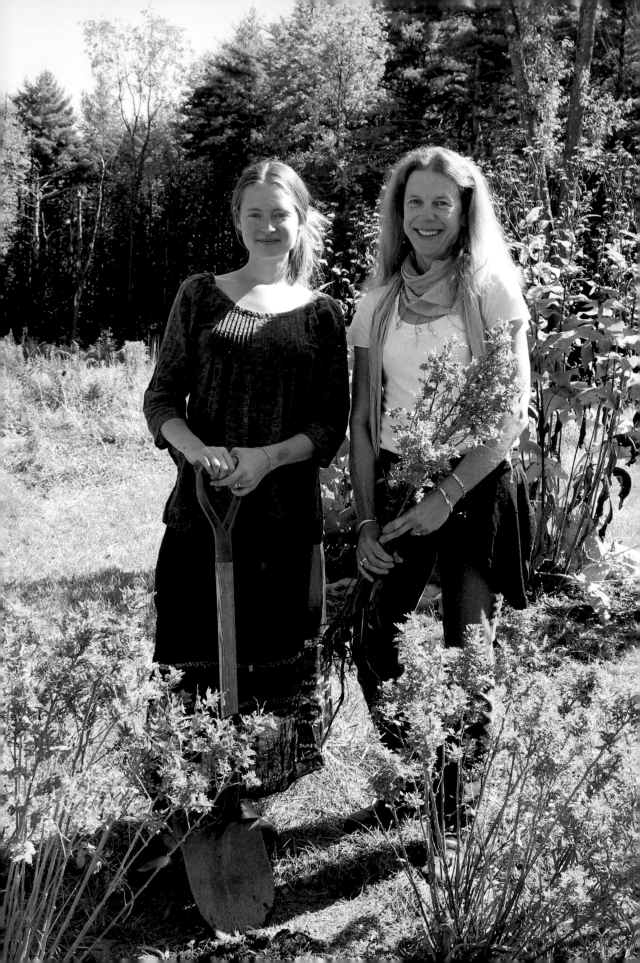

ABOUT THE AUTHORS

Dede's Journey from Patient to Gardener

I have Crohn's disease, which is a disease of the small intestine and is not curable, according to the Western medicine world. I surprised my doctor and have had eleven years of clinical remission after a bowel resection in 2006. These years have been filled with hope and health, though it is easy to fall into despair when the doctors tell you that your disease has gone from nonexistent to "severe."

Rather than saying, "Woe is me," and spending time feeling sad and useless (I did a lot of that, believe me), I decided to take action, and try to live the words of the Dalai Lama:

Scientists say that a healthy mind is a major factor for a healthy body, His Holiness said. If you're serious about your health, think and take most concern for your peace of mind. That's very, very important.

That said, I am on my way to health—no time to sit on my cushion meditating (I do that daily for a few minutes still); rather, I need to stay focused and take care of my body: better food, sleep, stress relief, education, awareness, team building, satisfying work, making money enough to live on, giving back to my community and the world . . . working for peace, justice, and environmental sustainability.

In the last few years, I began to grow some of my own vegetables, and I joined a local Community Support Agriculture (CSA) farm share. After realizing how easy it was to join the group (and I received a half-price share because we didn't need the family-sized one since my kids are grown now), I planned my own vegetable garden a few years ago. I worked with a naturopathic doctor, who prescribed many herbs, like turmeric, to help me keep inflammation in the small intestine at a low level. The next phase was for me to plan and grow my own herbs at home—there is nothing more satisfying than growing fresh herbs—the fresh smell in the kitchen is enough to please even those olfactory-challenged among us!

This new lifestyle is giving me strength and vitality. It is not for everyone—and I always tell people you must proceed with a doctor's knowledge, for Crohn's and the other auto-immune disease of the large intestine, ulcerative colitis, can be serious, even fatal, if not managed correctly. Since Crohn's is persistent, and they say cannot be cured, I needed to work with a naturopathic physician, along with my gastroenterologist.

I see a growing respect on both sides of the medicinal world —and I expect our book to help people even more.

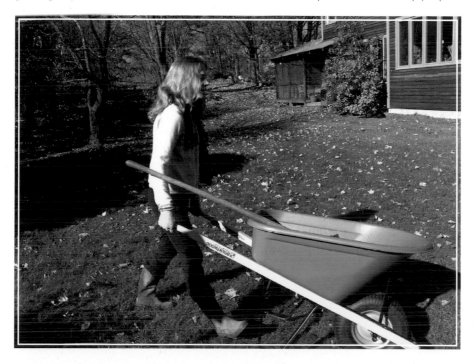

Alyssa's Herbalism Story

I suppose it began when I was old enough to play in the woods—around 4 years old. I spent most of my days in the woods and fields around my house. I grew up in the country, in southern Vermont. I always have had a close relationship with nature and, from a very young age, gardening as well. I helped my dad in the garden as soon as I could walk—well, sometimes not really helping, but trying to! Thinking back to those days, it was a simple life, a life of wonder and beauty, often by myself—as I am an only child—and sometimes with beloved friends, frolicking through the woods picking plants and creating magic.

There were times in my middle and later childhood years that I didn't seem to commune with the plants and nature so much, but it was rooted in me, I never forgot.

The next big part of my journey, which led me directly to the love for medicinal plants that I hold today, was college. I went to an amazing place—Sterling College, up in the hills of Northern Vermont. I went there with an interest in the environment, but wasn't initially clear on what my main interest within that would be. It became obvious within my first year, that agriculture was very exciting to me, and that I wanted to be a farmer in some capacity. In my second year, I traveled to western New York and worked on a 10-acre organic vegetable farm, 60 hours a week. It was hard work with many vegetables to sling. It was so rewarding, but through that experience, and a few others working with vegetables and fruits, it was clear that I most likely wouldn't pursue a life in this work.

Around the time after working in the vegetable fields, I took a trip over to Hyde Park, Vermont, which was a half hour from my school. There I toured the Zack Woods Herb Farm. A spark was ignited in me then that is still burning to this day. All the systems seemed to make sense to me, the growing of these plants that you could dry and preserve, and use later . . . the beauty and fragrance . . . the opportunity to know these plants, create remedies, and help myself and others feel better. It all made sense to me that day.

My friend and I took on the job of campus herbalists for the next year or so, planting an herb garden, harvesting herbs from the wild, and making simple remedies for our fellow students and teachers. That was so much fun!

Also during my college years I went to the Big Island of Hawaii and apprenticed with Barbarah Fahs of Hi'iaka's Healing Herb Garden, which was comprised of native Hawaiian herbs, as well as Western herbs. We tended the 1-acre intensely planted garden, made many medicines, and sold them through her little cottage shop, and the farmer's market. This Hawaii experience was one of the most memorable of my life, instilling deeply my love for working with and sharing plant medicine. Thoughts like "I could definitely do this for the rest of my life" abounded during that time—and have ever since!

After college a friend and I started up a small herb business called Rising Rhythm Herbs, which was focused on growing herbs for our community, really fun formulas, many of them aphrodisiac medicines, bundles of fresh herbs, and freshly brewed teas for farmer's markets and festivals. We dove into the the world of wholesaling, as well as online retail. This continued and thrived as a part of my life for about 10 years. Throughout part of this time I immersed myself in the study of Ayurvedic medicine, incorporating the parts I love from the ancient healing system into my life.

In 2011, I joined forces with several other health practitioners who were friends of mine to start a worker-owned health cooperative—the Brattleboro Holistic Health Center. I managed and made medicines for the Apothecary.

In the past few years and presently, I have a full apothecary on my homestead where I see clients, make medicine, and offer retreats, learning groups, and apprenticeships. I continue learning and deepening my practice through the principles of vitalism and am heavily focused on customizing remedies that address the root causes of peoples health issues. Find all info and contact at: www.vitalvesselherbs.love.

Throughout these years, I have been tending my herb garden, wild-crafting from my land and the surrounding forests and fields, making medicine for my family and friends, raising my two daughters with my husband while living in community, and trying to appreciate all that I have to be grateful for in this life, all that is sacred.

Herbs give me hope in the world, they empower me, remind me that I can heal and help others. They truly comfort me in times of darkness, and illness, and generally make my life joyous, radiant, and fulfilling.

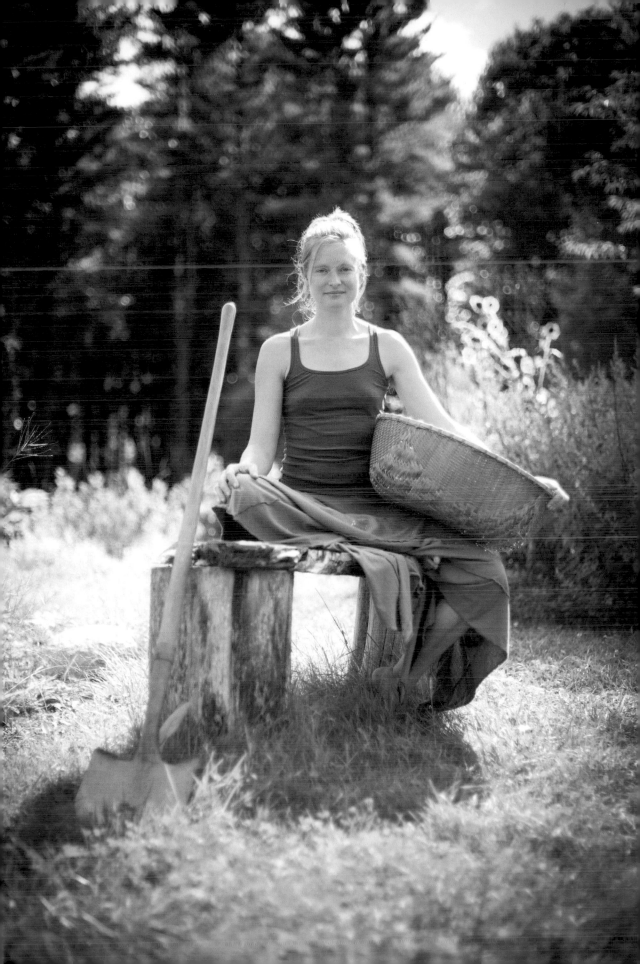

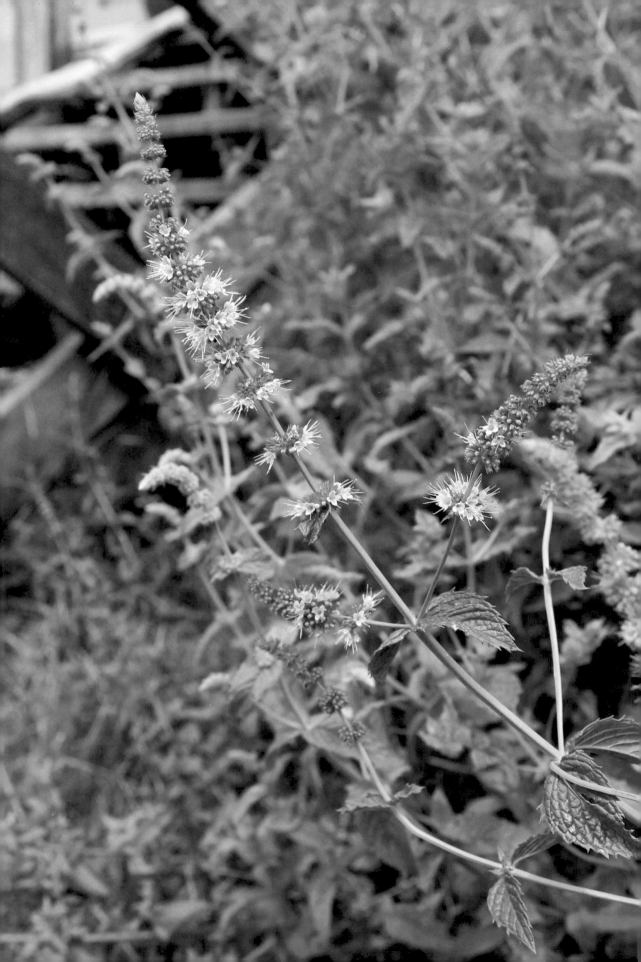